Lanchester Library

WITHDRAWN

THE EPIDEMIOLOGY OF
NEUROLOGICAL DISORDERS

THE EPIDEMIOLOGY OF NEUROLOGICAL DISORDERS

Edited by

Christopher Martyn
MRC Environmental Epidemiology Unit
Southampton General Hospital, UK

RAC Hughes
Professor of Neurology, UMDS
London, UK

© BMJ Books 1998
BMJ Books is an imprint of the BMJ Publishing Group

All rights reserved. No part of this publication may be reproduced,
stored in a retrieval system, or transmitted, in any form or by any
means, electronic, mechanical, photocopying, recording and/or
otherwise, without the prior written permission of the publishers.

First published in 1998
by BMJ Books, BMA House, Tavistock Square,
London WC1H 9JR

British Library Cataloguing in Publication Data

A catalogue record for this book is available from the British Library

ISBN 0-7279-1149-X

Po 01660
4.3.98

Coventry University

Typeset, printed and bound by
Latimer Trend & Company Ltd, Plymouth

Contents

Contributors

Dr Yoav Ben-Shlomo
Department of Social Medicine
University of Bristol
Bristol, UK

Dr Mary Cannon
Department of Psychiatry
University of Nottingham
Nottingham, UK

Professor Alastair Compston
Department of Neurology
Addenbrookes Hospital
Cambridge, UK

Professor Bryan Jennett
Institute of Neurological Sciences
Southern General Hospital
Glasgow, UK

Dr Peter Jones
Department of Psychiatry
University of Nottingham
Nottingham, UK

Professor Kay-Tee Khaw
Department of Clinical Gerontology
University of Cambridge
Cambridge, UK

Dr Neil Robertson
University of Cambridge Neurology Unit
Addenbrooke's Hospital
Cambridge, UK

Dr Gustavo Román
San Antonio
Texas, USA

Dr Josemir Sander
Epilepsy Research Group
Institute of Neurology
London, UK

Professor Simon Shorvon
Epilepsy Research Group
Institute of Neurology
London, UK

Dr Cornelia van Duijn
Department of Epidemiology and Statistics
Erasmus University Medical School
Rotterdam, The Netherlands

Dr Derick Wade
Rivermead Rehabilitation Centre
Abingdon Road
Oxford, UK

Preface

Traditionally, neurologists, neurosurgeons and psychiatrists relied on careful observation of individual cases to delineate syndromes and diseases. Recently they have become more uneasy about the limitations of a view obtained only from the bedside or outpatient clinic. They have seized opportunities for studying diseases in populations, rather than in hospitals, to give a very different picture. A wider epidemiological perspective contributes not only to a more profound understanding of the causes and natural history of disease but provides information that leads to better treatment. Not long ago, few epidemiological studies in neurology went much beyond estimates of the prevalence of disease. Now, many studies show that the repertoire of epidemiological methods has much to offer the neuroscientist.

This volume gathers together a series of articles that first appeared in the *Journal of Neurology, Neurosurgery and Psychiatry* and contains many examples of the value of such methods. Professor Bryan Jennett shows how knowledge of the causes of head injuries and their relative frequency informs both the clinical management of individual cases and the provision of neurosurgical services. Derick Wade takes an epidemiological standpoint to argue the need for a new way of thinking about what determines disability. Peter Jones and Mary Cannon in their chapter on schizophrenia show, amongst other things, how longitudinal studies can supply information unobtainable in other ways. Epidemiological investigations have some notable neurological successes to their credit. A recent instance is the case-control studies that demonstrated the importance of Campylobacter infection in the aetiology of Guillain-Barré syndrome. But there are some failures too. Yoav Ben-Shlomo documents the lack of progress in identifying the causes of Parkinson's disease and offers some explanations. Multiple sclerosis is another disease where, despite years of endeavour, epidemiology has faltered. Alastair Compston is caustic that so much activity should have discovered so little of real importance. He suggests that genetic epidemiology will be more fruitful. As Cornelia van Duijn describes, the combination of genetics and epidemiology has certainly advanced our understanding of Alzheimer's disease.

The series of articles in the *JNNP* was intended neither as an introduction to epidemiological methods nor as a systematic review of epidemiological studies in neurological and psychiatric disease. Our main aim was to encourage the widespread and growing interest in neuroepidemiology. We wanted to show the immediate relevance of the subject for clinicians; how knowledge gained from population-based research can influence and improve the everyday practice of neurology and psychiatry. The series had another purpose too. It drew attention to the many areas that had yet to be studied. Epidemiology is a field in which clinicians can make a unique contribution to neurosciences. We hope that gathering the articles together into a single volume will be useful and that it will stimulate clinicians to collaborate with epidemiologists in advancing understanding of causation and management of diseases of the nervous system.

Christopher Martyn
Richard Hughes

1 Parkinson's disease

YOAV BEN-SHLOMO

- Epidemiological studies of Parkinson's disease are hampered by difficulties in case definition, identification of relevant exposure periods and deficiencies in routinely collected data.
- There is little geographical variation in the rates of Parkinson's disease in Europe, but the disease seems to be less common in China and West Africa.
- There are few consistent findings regarding environmental exposures and risk of Parkinson's disease. But there is some evidence to implicate pesticides, head injury and low intake of some vitamins.
- The inverse relation between smoking and Parkinson's disease is found repeatedly in case-control and cohort studies.
- The lack of a social class gradient in risk of Parkinson's disease is difficult to reconcile with either a neurotoxic or infective hypothesis of aetiology.

... the writer will repine at no censure which the precipitate publication of mere conjectural suggestions may incur: but shall think himself fully rewarded by having excited the attention of those, who may point out the most appropriate means of relieving a tedious and most distressing malady.

JAMES PARKINSON[1]

It is almost 180 years since James Parkinson described his series of patients with what is now known as Parkinson's disease. His own astute clinical observations were unable to discern any obvious aetiology. "On the subject indeed of remote causes, no satisfactory account has yet been obtained from any of the sufferers."[1] He noted an indulgence in alcohol, lying on damp ground, and the possibility of trauma. He also reported the occupations of three of his patients; one was a gardener, another a sailor, and the third a magistrate. Even in 1817, the disease affected a broad social range of society. We have made some progress in elucidating the cause of Parkinson's disease over this period but this has been limited. For instance, the role of trauma in the aetiology of Parkinson's disease remains uncertain and disputed.[2-4] Epidemiological research has steadily increased, particularly over the past 10 years, and more research has been directed towards analytical rather than just descriptive studies. More recently, work in the area of genetic epidemiology[5] has begun and researchers are now focusing on both molecular and environmental risk factors. This review interprets the existing evidence and provides a personal view on what we definitively know about the epidemiology of Parkinson's disease, what remains speculative, and what questions remain to be answered.

Problems facing a neuroepidemiologist

It is important to appreciate the problems and limitations faced by neuroepidemiologists attempting to study Parkinson's disease. These drawbacks help to explain some of the rather inconclusive and often contradictory findings between studies.

Study Design

Most analytical studies use a case-control approach. This is because Parkinson's disease is relatively rare. Any prospective study needs to have a large sample size to generate sufficient cases for analysis. The combined alumni cohorts of Harvard and Pennsylvania colleges consisted of 50 000 people and only generated 160 cases.[6] Older cohorts will be more efficient in terms of statistical power. Case-control studies, although far more practical, are more prone to bias. Particularly problematic is the recruitment of control subjects and the measurement of putative exposures. Associations must be treated with some caution and if possible verified using either historical data or a cohort design.

Case Definition

The case definition for Parkinson's disease is based on clinical criteria. Only two thirds of potential cases of Parkinson's disease recruited directly from primary care may truly have the disease as validated by postmortem diagnosis.[7] Prevalence studies from various countries have shown that potential cases will include patients with benign essential tremor, dementia, and cerebro-vascular disease.[8-10] In Aberdeen, 15% of potential cases were excluded after specialist examination.[8] A clinical diagnosis by a neurologist or geriatrician is also limited. The United Kingdom Parkinson's Disease Society Brain Bank data have shown that the predictive value of an expert diagnosis is only around 75%.[11] The use of stricter clinical criteria can improve the predictive value but this is at the cost of excluding more genuine cases and is therefore only really of value for therapeutic trials rather than epidemiological studies.[12] The use of complex investigations, such as PET, is not suitable for large epidemiological studies. The result of including other disorders as well as true cases of Parkinson's disease in a study will depend on the relation between these diseases and the exposures of interest. If this is no different to that found for Parkinson's disease, the results will not be biased. It is more reasonable to assume that they do not share the same aetiological factors. In this case, misclassification will bias the results towards the null; it will be harder to show a relation between exposure and disease, even if it truly exists.

Measurement of Exposure

The measurement of exposure is also problematic. It is unclear as to when in the lifecourse an exposure may be important (fig 1.1). Clinical symptoms are thought to start once cell loss has

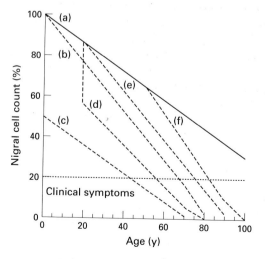

Figure 1.1   Nigral cell loss: possible periods during the lifecourse for the role of an environmental factor. Cell loss is shown at a constant rate for simplicity; see text for details. (Modified from Langston[17].)

3

reached a threshold level of 70% to 80%. Normal age-related cell loss (a) is thought not to result in disease unless current life expectancy is prolonged. A genetic model might propose that cell loss from birth occurred in some people at a faster than normal rate (b) due to "aging genes".[13] Intrauterine events, such as infection or placental abnormalities,[14 15] might result in a person being born with a depleted cell count and normal age related loss (c) would ensure that disease would appear in later life. This developmental model has been proposed to explain the discordance rate seen for monozygotic twins.[15] Environmental factors could act through an acute mechanism—for example, a head injury (d) destroying a finite number of cells—followed by normal age related loss (two stage hypothesis).[16] Alternatively a low level chronic exposure (e)—for example, a diet relatively deficient in antioxidants—may simply act by slightly accelerating the rate of cell death. Finally an acute event—for example, exposure to a toxic chemical—may act by triggering cell death which results in a cascade of events and accelerated cell death (f). This final model would suggest that a long latency period may not be essential for disease aetiology and would focus attention on later life. Most people believe that a long latency period for Parkinson's disease is most likely.[17-19] However, pathological data challenge the hypothesis that age related cell loss on top of an external insult is important.[20] It is also possible that causation is heterogenous and that any one of the various models might operate in different persons to produce cell loss and this would be clinically indistinguishable.

Recently, the temporal profile of neurodegeneration in Parkinson's disease has been compared by various mathematical models to distinguish between different patterns of cell loss.[21] Several important, and possibly questionable, assumptions had to be made to enable the calculations to be performed. The empirical data seemed to be compatible with both an "event" that kills some neurons and reduces the life expectancy of others and a "process" which continuously kills healthy neurons at a constant rate. It did, however, exclude a process which resulted in either an accelerating or decelerating cell death.

Most exposures are measured by subjective recall. This has two problems: low impact exposure, such as past diet, is likely to be poorly recalled by both cases and controls (non-differential misclassification). This will dilute any true relation and lead to erroneously concluding that there is no relation. High impact exposures might be differentially recalled by cases and not controls, particularly if there is pre-existing knowledge of a possible link between the exposure and disease. For example, a previous head injury might be more salient in the minds of patients than in controls, as they may link the trauma with their neurological disease (recall bias).

Geographical Patterns

International comparisons have in the past relied on mortality rates adjusted for demographic differences between countries. Early findings showed a sevenfold to eightfold variation in mortality rates[22][23] suggesting an important role for environmental factors as well as possible genetic differences. Mortality rates are susceptible to variations in diagnosis, survival, and certification practice, which could produce large artefactual differences. This is best illustrated by the fivefold mortality differences between Scotland and Japan.[22] However, there is little difference in the prevalence rates for patients between 60 and 69 years of age, when underascertainment should be less problematic (Scotland 254/100 000[8]; Japan 245/100 000).[9] More complex approaches differentiate between "multisource" prevalence studies, which rely on the complete identification of patients with a pre-existing diagnosis, and "population based" surveys which screen a total defined population identifying both pre-existing and new cases.[24] The population based survey method is particularly important for developing countries because of limited medical services or for communities in which there may be differential access to health care. For example, differential access to health care for ethnic minorities is well recognised in the United States[25] and in the Copiah county study, more previously undiagnosed black patients (58%) than white patients (32%) were found.[26] The population based survey method ·also enables more valid comparisons between studies as ascertainment is more standardised than conventional multisource studies. Unfortunately, as the prevalence rates are usually based on relatively few cases they are less robust, with wide confidence intervals.

Age adjusted prevalence rates suggest that a threefold difference may exist, with Libya (57/100 000) at one end and Iceland (182/100 000) at the other.[24] Prevalence rates are also susceptible to differences in diagnosis and survival. Artefactual differences can be reduced by limiting the comparison to European countries with good healthcare systems, using incidence rates as these are independent of differences in survival, and comparing rates for subjects under 70 years, in whom underascertainment should not be important.[27] These results (table 1.1) suggest threefold variations, but this is reduced to less than twofold (80%) if Iceland is excluded. No obvious geographical pattern emerges, and the rates for Denmark and Holland are more similar to Sardinia than rates from Ferrara, Italy. Community door to door studies suggest that prevalence rates (fig 1.2) are fairly similar between both developed and some developing countries except for China and west Africa. A recent pilot study from Taiwan (not shown in fig 1.2) found much higher rates than in China, even though it was carried out in a rural area.[28] This suggests that black persons in America and Chinese in Taiwan have higher rates of disease than their counterparts in west Africa or China. Environmental factors may thus be more important than racial factors in explaining these variations.[26]

A recent report on the prevalence of Lewy bodies in brains from Nigerians examined at postmortem has shown similar rates to those in western populations.[29] Assuming that incidental Lewy bodies reflect preclinical disease, this finding supports the notion that the propensity to develop Parkinson's disease is universal. It also supports the role of environmental factor(s), as it is still necessary to explain why some Afro-Americans go on to develop clinical disease whereas their African counterparts remain asymptomatic.[30]

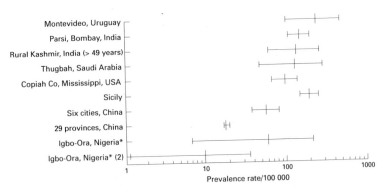

Figure 1.2   Age adjusted prevalence rates/100 000 from door to door surveys. * *Indicates crude prevalence and not age adjusted. The study by Tison et al[66] from Gironde, France is not shown. (Data amended from Zhang and Roman.[24])*

Table 1.1 Age specific incidence rates per 100 000 for Parkinson's disease from selected European studies

Country (period)	Rates per age group							Relative rates* (95% CIs)
	30–39	40–49	50–59	60–69	70–79	80–89	50–69	
Iceland (1954–63)	1·4	5·6	32·9	97·2	136·2	69·2	61·3	2·75 (2·31–3·27)
Southwest Finland (1968–70)	0·7	2·6	19·8	62·3	92·6	47·9	40·1	1·80 (1·46–2·21)
Ferrara, Italy (1967–87)	0·7	7·2	25·1	49·6	45·8	1·1	35·9	1·61 (1·40–1·86)
Aarhus, Denmark (1967–70)	0·0	1·0	15·8	39·8	58·5	28·1	26·8	1·20 (0·90–1·60)
Netherlands (1983–5)	0·0	0·0	14·5	25·7	79·3	117·2	19·5	0·88 (0·54–1·42)
Sardinia, Italy	1·3	7·1	26·4	18·0	4·3	0·0	22·3	1·00

*Relative rate for 50–69 years compared with Sardinia, Italy.
Data taken from de Pedro-Cuesta.[27]

Comment

It is clear that Parkinson's disease is found throughout the world, but is less common in some countries such as China and Africa. This may reflect racial differences in genetic susceptibility or the absence of specific environmental factors related to industrialisation. In China there is some evidence to support the role of industrialisation as residing in a village residence was seen to be protective.[31] There is a need for further migrant studies to elucidate the role of environmental factors.[32] Across Europe there is relatively little variation, and what there is may be explained by methodological differences. Current standardised population based prevalence surveys will determine whether these differences are artefactual. The surprisingly high rates seen in Iceland may be idiosyncratic or reflect a higher degree of ascertainment when surveying a small population.[33] Analysis of more recent drug utilisation data for Iceland supports this finding.[34] Further work should confirm this observation and explore possible reasons, be they genetic or environmental.

Temporal patterns

Mortality rates

Descriptions of what might have been Parkinson's disease existed well before the nineteenth century. The ancient ayurvedic literature (4500–1000 BC) of India describes an illness "kampavata" consisting of tremor and akinesia.[35] Analysis of temporal trends have mostly relied on long term patterns in mortality rates. Studies from several different countries have all shown similar patterns of mortality over time: the United States,[36-38] United Kingdom,[39-42] Ireland,[43] Italy,[44] Norway,[45] Denmark,[36] and Japan.[46] Mortality rates for both men and women have shown increases for older age groups (> 75 years), and a decline for younger age groups (< 65 years). These patterns are remarkably consistent and predate the widespread introduction of levodopa in the 1970s. There are several possible explanations for these patterns.

1. Awareness, diagnosis, and certification of Parkinson's disease, particularly in elderly patients, may have increased over time. This might explain some of the increase seen for older patients but is unlikely to explain the rise seen before

the 1970s. It is unlikely to explain the differential increase in mortality seen for men compared with women.[38] White men over 80 showed a 100% greater increase than women when comparing mortality changes between 1962 and 1984. This is unlikely to reflect diagnosis or treatment and could reflect occupational risk factors.[38] This pattern has also been seen in data from England and Wales (unpublished personal observation).

2. Levodopa treatment may have increased survival resulting in a shift of the age specific mortality curve to the right by about five years.[36] There is some evidence to suggest that the initial introduction of levodopa treatment may have delayed death.[47] However, more recent survival cohorts[48][49] suggest that mortality from Parkinson's disease compared with that of the general population has not altered to a large degree from the pre-levodopa days.[50] There has been a secular increase in life expectancy for the whole population, so that a patient with Parkinson's disease today would expect to live longer like anyone else in the population.

3. There may have been a genuine change in the incidence of disease:

(a) The incidence of disease in elderly people may have increased because of a reduction in heart disease and stroke mortality and hence a decline in competing causes of death.[51] If the risk of Parkinson's disease was also associated with heart disease or stroke, a reduction in deaths from heart disease would selectively increase the pool of potential subjects who could develop Parkinson's disease. Only one study has shown such an association[49] and this has not been replicated.[52] If these diseases are independent of each other, then whereas a reduction of heart disease will increase the absolute number of cases of Parkinson's disease, it will not alter the age specific rates.

(b) There has been a decrease in the incidence of disease in young age groups due to a decrease in environmental exposures.[37]

(c) The divergence of age specific mortality rates reflects a cohort effect due to a self limiting exposure, such as the encephalitis lethargica epidemic.[53][54] Such a hypothesis would predict an increase in mortality as "exposed" cohorts aged but a decline in the mortality of younger

9

age groups who would have been born after the exposure. As these later unexposed cohorts reached old age there would be a subsequent reduction in mortality for all ages. There have been several attempts to examine the cohort hypothesis using mortality data.[40 41 43] Plotting mortality rates by birth cohort suggests excess mortality for cohorts born between 1875 and 1895. Standardised mortality ratios for those aged 30–50 in 1920 in England and Wales were raised compared with those born earlier or later.[40] More recent multivariate modelling methods have been developed to disentangle age, period, and cohort effects.[55] Initial analyses using these methods support these findings for both England and Wales and United States data (C Martyn, personal communication). Despite these complex methods, there is still an essential problem that cohorts born after the epidemic from the mid-1930s are still relatively young (< 65 years) and have not reached the age when mortality rates have been shown to be increasing. The cohort hypothesis is also unlikely to explain the differential mortality increase seen for men (see above) as there was little difference in encephalitis lethargica mortality rates for men and women.[56]

Incidence Rates

Incidence rates are far superior to mortality rates, but are still potentially biased by temporal trends in consulting behaviour and doctor diagnosis. Data from Rochester, Minnesota are unique in covering a long period (1935–79).[57–59] The annual incidence rate has increased from 11·4/100 000 in 1935–44 to 18·2/100 000 between 1967 and 1979. The age adjusted rates have remained fairly constant over the past 30 years.[24] Age adjusted rates can mask heterogeneity in age specific patterns as rates in older age groups could increase whereas those in younger groups decreased leaving the adjusted rate unchanged. The use of different age groupings in the two previous publications[58 59] makes it impossible to compare the age specific rates over this entire period. Comparing 1945–54 with 1955–66, it does seem that the rate for patients aged between 40–69 has decreased whereas that for those over 70 years has increased.[60]

Comment

Temporal data are limited and difficult to interpret. Mortality rates among elderly people have increased substantially but the interpretation of this finding is controversial. The most reliable data to answer this question come from Rochester, Minnesota. A reanalysis of the Rochester data including more recent data between 1980 and 1995 is essential to help us discriminate between various competing hypotheses.

Individual risk factors

Sociodemographic factors: age, sex, and social class

The risk of developing Parkinson's disease increases as a person gets older. But, it is unclear whether the increase in risk is continuous or eventually declines for the oldest age groups. The first pattern would favour the notion of "aging-related" degeneration as has been argued for Alzheimer's dementia.[61] Multisource prevalence studies suggest that prevalence rates generally fall for the oldest age groups (table 1.1). It is likely that older subjects are less likely to present for medical attention, are more difficult to diagnose, and even when under residential care may be missed.[62] Population based studies consistently show that prevalence rates increase continuously in an exponential fashion.[26 63-66] Because broad age groups are used to calculate the age specific rates, it is possible that these studies could mask a flattening of the age curve. However, the study from Gironde, France calculated rates for five year age groups between 65 and older than 90 years and also found an exponential rise.[66]

Most studies support an excess of male to female cases. The average ratio of male to female standardised rates is 1·35 from prevalence studies and 1·31 from incidence studies, but the range is wide.[24] This excess is seen for both multisource and population based studies. Hospital based studies may be misleading, as there is evidence that the survival of women recruited from hospitals is worse than men and hence will bias the results in favour of increasing the prevalence of men compared with women.[49]

Adult social class is a variable often measured in epidemiological studies[67] as it is so strongly related to many diseases,[68] and is often used as a confounding variable when examining other exposures. American studies tend to use a

11

classification based on years of education or income, whereas European studies are more likely to use an occupation based classification.[69] As a variable it is non-specific, and acts as a proxy marker for many other exposures such as smoking, diet, obesity, occupational exposures, sanitary conditions, overcrowding, risk of infection, income, etc. Many potential risk factors are distributed in a graded fashion by socioeconomic class. Showing a gradient in disease by socioeconomic class is often not very helpful as it fails to indicate which one of the many potential exposures is of importance. However, the lack of a gradient is of relevance as it challenges conventional hypotheses. For example, if it is speculated that Parkinson's disease is the result of a chemical exposure, it is likely that such an exposure would be greater for manual rather than non-manual jobs, unless the chemical is commonly found in the domestic home environment. Similarly, risk of infection will be associated with crowding, sanitary conditions, and hence socioeconomic class.

Mortality data from the United Kingdom show no social class gradient for deaths between 20–64 years. For older ages there is a gradient with higher ratios in social class I and II than IV and V.[70] However, proportional mortality ratios are influenced by the strong social class gradient for other more common causes of death, which would artefactually increase the proportion of mortality from Parkinson's disease in higher social classes.[71] More reliable data can be obtained from case-control studies. Unfortunately, few studies have either examined or reported the results for adult social class and none have reported parental social class, which would reflect childhood living conditions.

Almost every study has failed to show any relation with years of education.[72-75] One study which did show that cases were better educated[76] failed to adjust for age or sex, two important confounders as controls were both older and were more likely to be women. Similarly, a study of early onset Parkinson's disease showed an initial twofold increased risk associated with having completed high school graduation, but this was almost completely attenuated after adjustment for smoking habit and other variables.[77] A case-control study with discordant twin pairs suggested that cases were less likely to be manual workers but this was not significant (odds ratio 0·50; 95% confidence interval (95% CI) 0·10–2·23).[78] Only one prospective study has reported social class and again found no relation.[79] Farming has been examined as a specific occupation with a possible raised risk. Some[75 80 81] but not all studies[82 83] have shown an increased risk. This could relate to pesticide use or other exposures that are more common in rural areas (see later).

Comment

Parkinson's disease is more common among older subjects and men. Limited evidence suggests that risk increases continuously with age. Further evidence is required to test the "aging related" hypothesis by focusing on population surveys of elderly people. It is important to determine why men have an increased risk compared with women. This could be related to smoking behaviour or other toxic exposures. Most case-control studies match cases and controls by sex, and are unable to examine the odds ratio associated with sex before and after adjustment for other risk factors. A population based case-control study, which does not match subjects by sex, would be useful to clarify this issue. There seems to be little social class or educational gradient. If anything, the risk seems increased with higher socioeconomic class or more years of education. The lack of a gradient is surprising as exposures to toxic agents, infectious agents, etc are likely to differ by social class. Adult social class is moderately correlated with parental social class but over the past 60 years there has been upward social mobility. Exposures acting in childhood may be more relevant than adult factors and future studies need to examine childhood circumstances by collecting data on parental social class as well as other childhood variables.

Specific exposures

Many potential exposures have been cited as possible risk factors for Parkinson's disease. These can broadly be divided into three groups: toxic exposures, infectious exposures, and a heterogenous group of miscellaneous exposures. Table 1.2 lists some of the studies that have investigated these exposures. Cohort studies provide the most robust observational data.

Toxic exposures

The report that 1-methyl-4-phenyl-1,2,5,6-tetrahydropyridine (MPTP) has neurotoxic effects in humans[114] has led to the hunt

Table 1.2 Relationship between environmental risk factors and Parkinson's disease according to study design

Risk factor	Ecological studies		Case control studies			Cohort studies	
	Increased risk	No relationship	Increased risk	Decreased risk	No relationship	Decreased risk	No relationship
Toxic exposures:							
Pesticides, herbicides	84		75,77,80,81,85		74,82,83,86,87		
Solvents					78,86		
Mercury	89		88		86		
Industrial residence			31		90		
Infectious exposures:							
Shingles					78		
Measles					72		6
Chicken pox					72	6	6
Mumps					72		
Influenza	14						6
Whooping cough	34	91					6
							104
Miscellaneous exposures:							
Smoking			94,105–107	72,74,77,78, 92–98	76,80,88,99, 100	79,90, 101–103	108
Personality			74,95		77,81		
Head trauma			80,82,83,85,87, 88		74,77,81,90		
Rural residence	84		82,83,87,90	31	109		
Well water			80		31,74,85,109		
Raw vegetables			77	85,110,111	76,80,88,98	112	
Dietary antioxidants				90,100	113		79
Alcohol					98,100	79	
Coffee							

If a study has a non-significant result, it has been classified as showing no relationship even if the results are in the same direction as other studies.

for a more commonly occurring environmental toxin. The validity of using the MPTP model to generate clues relating to idiopathic Parkinson's disease is generally thought to be reasonable.[115] Paraquat is similar in structure to MPTP[116] and therefore most attention has focused on herbicides and pesticides, although other toxic compounds, such as manganese and mercury, which are known to have neurological effects, have also been examined. An early ecological study from Canada showed a positive relation between a rural area with the greatest pesticide usage and both Parkinson's disease mortality and drug utilisation levels.[84] Case-control studies can be divided into those that show an association[75 77 80 81 85] and those that do not.[74 82 83 86 87] Several possibilities exist to explain these discrepant results. Most of the studies that show an association, suggest a threefold increased risk associated with pesticide use. A weak study may have insufficient power to detect such a risk and would lead to a spurious negative finding (type II error). However, several of the negative studies were sufficiently large to have significantly detected such an increased risk.[83 87] For example, the Kansas study was sufficiently powerful to detect a twofold increased risk.[83] Most of the studies have measured occupational pesticide exposures[75 83] but some have included domestic exposure.[74 80] Recall bias is unlikely to explain this association as there is no reason that it should operate in some but not all studies given the similarity of their populations. Empirical evidence suggests that differential recall for pesticides between cases and controls is not a serious consideration.[117] Studies that show an increased risk with pesticides also tend to be the same studies with an increased risk for rural residence. This is to be expected as occupational pesticide use is likely to be more common in rural areas. An artefactual association between pesticides and Parkinson's disease could exist if "selection bias" resulted in an over-representation of rural cases compared with rural controls (see section on rural residence for detailed discussion). However, in some studies the association with pesticide use was present[75] despite no association with rural residence[109] and vice versa.[83] The study from Calgary, Canada[75 109] is particularly impressive as its design should have minimised any selection bias and it also obtained detailed occupational histories. One possibility is that pesticides differ between studies and only some types show an association with Parkinson's disease. However, this explanation is unlikely as most of these studies

15

cover a similar period and examine populations in North America.

Cross sectional data show an association between exposure to organophosphate pesticides and subtle differences in both cognitive processing and depression.[118] Depression has been shown to be common in Parkinson's disease and may predate clinical symptoms.[119 120] It is not clear whether these results have any relevance to the pathophysiology of Parkinson's disease. As this study was cross sectional, it is uncertain whether such subtle cognitive differences may not have existed before the exposure. Only limited data are available on occupational cohorts. The "Iowa 65+ rural health study" showed that farmers, either still working or retired, were less likely to have Parkinson's disease compared with other rural controls.[121] No information was provided, however, as regards their pesticide exposure and smoking habit was not taken into account.

The hypothesis that toxins are involved has been given much more credence by the recent discovery that patients with Parkinson's disease have relatively less effective detoxification systems.[122-126] This enhances the plausibility of the "ecogenetic" hypothesis that Parkinson's disease may result from the combination of an inherited susceptibility and an environmental toxin. If susceptibility is relatively rare—for example, the proportion of the general population with poor metaboliser status for debrisoquine is thought to be between 5% and 10%—the exposure may be common as most exposed subjects will not experience any adverse results. From an epidemiological perspective, a common exposure experienced by 80% or more of the general population will be much harder to detect and require far larger sample sizes. Studies will either need to be restricted to subjects with the susceptibility genes or must be able to test for interactions between genetic and exposure state.

The public health importance of pesticide use as a cause of Parkinson's disease is limited. Assuming a causal relation, the population attributable risk—that is, the percentage of all cases of Parkinson's disease that might be related to occupational pesticide use—is only around 10%, although this could vary between 2% and 25% (95% CI).[75] This estimate excludes non-occupational exposure, which is far more common although less intense. If some subjects are particularly susceptible to even low level exposure, then pesticides could pose a far more serious public health risk.

Infectious exposures

The notion that Parkinson's disease could be related to an infectious agent is far older and has existed since the recognition of postencephalitic parkinsonism. Other neurological diseases, such as subacute sclerosing panencephalitis, also provide an analogous model of disease related to latent infection. Whereas a toxic hypothesis has risen in popularity, an infectious hypothesis has declined and work examining infections is generally older.[6 14 34 72 78 91] Some authorities consider that "the disease is not of viral origin . . ."[127] and hence there is no further need to test this hypothesis. Indeed, the inconsistent seroepidemiological results[128 129] and failure to detect specific viral particles, inclusions, or antigens in brain necropsy material[130] suggest that pursuit of this hypothesis may be fruitless. However, several intriguing observations remain which require an answer. Serological analyses suggest, if anything, that serum antibody titres in cases of Parkinson's disease are often no different or lower than for controls. For example, titres for measles, rubella, herpes simplex 1, herpes simplex 2, mumps, and cytomegalovirus were all lower for patients, with the first three being statistically significant.[128] Although serological data are objective, they cannot identify the age at infection, which might be a more important predictor than infection itself.[34 131] Studies that have used subjective reporting of infections also show no significant differences between cases and controls, except for measles infection, which has been reported to be less frequent among college students who went on to to develop Parkinson's disease.[6] However, pertussis, chicken pox, and mumps infection also seem to be less common,[6 72] consistent with the serological results. It is unlikely that recall bias could explain this as these results were found in both retrospective and prospective studies. Simple misclassification would bias the results towards the null. A reduced frequency of childhood infections could be a chance phenomenon, but might relate to other factors, such as infection in very early life. One study suggested the possibility of "in utero" infection but this was based on ecological data[14] and failed to be replicated.[91] Alternatively, it may reflect variations in immune function or the possibility of confounding by another factor such as socioeconomic class or family size. The non-specificity of the results favours the role of a confounding factor, but this remains unresolved.

Miscellaneous exposures

Smoking and personality

The inverse relation between smoking and Parkinson's disease has been seen consistent for both case-control and cohort studies. Dorn, in one of the earliest smoking cohort studies,[101] was so surprised by the association that he sought and received confirmation from both Doll and Hill[103] and Hammond.[102] Some publications have failed to show a statistically significant association but in most studies the results have been in the same direction. The consistency of this finding in different populations and using different methods, makes it reasonable to exclude chance as an explanation for this association. Other possible explanations are

1. *Bias*—Subjects may biologically age at different rates due to genetic differences in the ability to repair cellular damage. Smoking may adversely affect DNA repair mechanisms and therefore smokers with less efficient mechanisms would be selectively eliminated (selective mortality). Older surviving cigarette smokers would have relatively more effective DNA repair mechanisms and would therefore be protected from developing either Parkinson's disease or Alzheimer's disease.[13] [132] This argument is flawed for two reasons.[133] Monozygotic twin pairs, when both twins are alive, still show the inverse association with smoking. Case-control studies using early onset cases show similar findings, even though selective mortality is unlikely to be of any importance for populations at this young age.

2. *Causality*—There are several biologically plausible reasons why smoking may protect or retard the development of Parkinson's disease. Hydrazine found in tobacco smoke protects mice from damage to nigrostriatal cells from MPTP.[134] Carbon monoxide or other factors in cigarette smoke may scavenge free radicals.[135] Smoking may have an effect on mitochondrial activity and oxidative damage.[136] Polyaromatic hydrocarbons in tobacco smoke may induce cytochrome *P-450* enzymes and lead to increased metabolism of xenobiotics.[137] If smoking did in fact alter the rate of nigral cell death it could be predicted that smokers who developed Parkinson's disease would both be older than non-smokers and would have a slower rate of disease

progression. Both of these predictions are refuted by empirical evidence.[98–100 138]

3. *Reverse causality*—Parkinson's disease makes people give up smoking as a secondary phenomenon. But the inverse association is still found if smoking habits are examined for a period before onset of clinical disease.[77 93] It is possible, however, that subtle changes in personality occur well before overt clinical disease as part of a more insidious onset. Such changes might affect smoking behaviour. Personality may therefore either act as a proxy marker of disease, or is a confounding variable unrelated to the disease process.

4. *Confounding*—There are premorbid personality differences associated with both the likelihood of becoming a smoker and continuing to smoke and other exposures/genes that are directly related to the risk of developing Parkinson's disease. Smokers seem to differ in personality traits from non-smokers and are more likely to be extrovert or exhibit type A behaviour.[139] Non-smokers have higher levels of shyness and defensiveness.[140] Similar personality differences may also determine alcohol consumption. Most studies show that patients with Parkinson's disease either are no different or have reduced alcohol consumption.[90 100] Patients with Parkinson's disease are reported to show personality changes, such as introvertism, that would make them less likely to be smokers.[94 105–107] We do not know, however, to what degree personality, such as being the more dominant twin,[107] could influence other risk factors, such as migration from rural to urban areas or reducing the risk of exposure to pesticides. Alternatively certain genes may influence both the tendency to smoke and the risk of developing Parkinson's disease. This argument has been suggested to explain the similar association found with Alzheimer's disease.[141]

Head trauma

Some studies have noted an excess risk of head trauma among patients with Parkinson's disease than among controls.[74 95 142] This association is usually doubted because of the likelihood that it reflects recall bias. One method to reduce this possible bias is to only measure severe head injuries, such as those resulting in loss of consciousness. Even though such events should be recalled equally well by both cases and controls, patients with Parkinson's disease still show an increased risk.[74] Another strategy to control for recall bias is to ask patients about their own "lay beliefs" as to what caused their disease.[143] Patients who report trauma as a possible cause can then be removed from the analysis to determine the degree of potential bias, although this might underestimate the true risk.[144] Only one study has examined a cohort of subjects with recorded head injuries and followed up their risk of Parkinson's disease. This study failed to find any increased risk but had a 30% probability of not detecting a twofold relative risk even if one existed.[108] Susceptibility to trauma, rather than severity itself may be more important. If head injury triggers a cascade of biological events that lead to cell death in only a few susceptible people, then it may be more difficult to detect an increased risk in a head injury cohort than in a case-control study.

Rural residence

It is paradoxical that industrialisation has been proposed to explain the differences in geographical prevalence rates between countries, yet within countries residing in a rural area has been noted to increase risk.[77 80 82 83 85 87 88] One of the first reports of such an association came from a Canadian series of 21 patients whose disease started under 41 years of age.[145] This series noted an excess of rural patients who had drunk well water. Rural residence, like social class, is a rather non-specific variable as it could simply be a proxy marker for various other exposures, such as well water consumption, farming, pesticide exposure, diet, contact with farm animals, or age at infection. Any genetic susceptibility to develop Parkinson's disease may also differ between urban and rural populations, as isolated rural populations might have a greater degree of inbreeding.

Some studies have suggested that rural exposure in early life is more important,[82] whereas others suggest that it is the total number of years.[80] This finding is not consistent, with some studies showing a decreased risk[31] or no significant risk.[74 77 81 90 109] Demographic variables, such as rural residence, are particularly sensitive to the method of recruiting controls[146] and the possibility of selection bias. Most studies recruit patients from neurology or movement disorder clinics based in urban centres. These specialist centres will often have a wide catchment area and see patients from both urban and rural areas. It is likely that elderly rural patients might be managed locally and not get referred on because of transport and access difficulties.[147] This is not likely for atypical, severe, and young patients and specialist clinics will have an overrepresentation of these.[148] Studies showing an increased risk (except one) selected controls from the hospital which recruited the cases. Controls were usually subjects with more common medical conditions such as heart or respiratory disease and would therefore be more likely to include local urban residents. Such a bias would artefactually increase the proportion of patients with Parkinson's disease from rural areas. The only exception[85] used spouses as controls. It is unclear whether spouses might be more or less likely to come from the same area as the patient and this would depend on the level of migration and mixing of urban and rural residents. Studies which failed to show any increased risk used various methods: "buddy" controls,[74] neurological clinic controls,[90] stratified sampling,[81] rheumatoid arthritis controls,[77] and population based control selection.[109] The use of buddy controls is not to be recommend as it may well result in overmatching.[149] Selecting patients from a specialist clinic may diminish selection bias but is also problematic especially if a single disease entity is chosen. Only the population based study ensured non-biased ascertainment of both cases and controls[109] and this study failed to show an association. In fact, rural residence in this study may have been associated with a decreased risk for those subjects not exposed to pesticides. As this study showed an increased risk for occupational pesticide use[75] and this would be more common in rural areas, the risk for rural subjects not exposed to pesticides must have been reduced so that the overall rural risk was not raised. It is interesting to note that the incidence study from Ferrara, Italy did observe a greater risk of Parkinson's disease in rural areas, but this was restricted to patients under 50 years and was not seen among housewives.[150]

Well water

Well water, like rural residence, has also been seen to be associated with Parkinson's disease. This is not surprising as the two exposures are closely correlated. Hence studies that show a relation between rural residence also tend to show a relation with well water and vice versa. The strong correlation between these two variables is evident in the Kansas case-control study. Well water had a significantly raised odds ratio of 1·7 with Parkinson's disease, but after adjusting for rural residence this was attenuated to 1·1.[83] One study specifically used factor analysis in an attempt to overcome the problems of excessive collinearity.[81] This is only a partial solution and does not overcome the problems of determining "independent" effects when measurement error is taken into account.[151] Designing studies that specifically break the confounding between two closely correlated exposures is better than using complex statistical methods, but is not always possible in reality.

Well water could act as a carrier of a potential toxin or as a vector for an infective agent. No relation has been noted, however, in either pesticides or heavy metal composition of water supply sampled for early onset cases and controls.[152] Other possible factors still need to be considered, such as the role of sulphur containing compounds. Patients with Parkinson's disease have reduced S-oxidation capacity and sulphate conjugation.[123] Alternatively, well water, like rural residence, may again be simply a proxy marker for another exposure which is more common in rural environments.

Dietary factors

Diet could play a part in the aetiology of Parkinson's disease. The rare disease of amyotrophic lateral sclerosis/parkinsonism-dementia, seen on the Islands of Guam and Rota, is thought to be due to a dietary toxin from the cycad plant,[153] which is not found in western diets. Diet is complex and it is difficult to quantify exposure.[154] Usually all subjects are exposed to the hypothesised causal factors and thus continuous variables need to be measured, often with a limited range of variation. Retrospective data are especially prone to inaccuracy and recall bias.[154] Recall of past diet in each case is seen to be strongly influenced by current dietary intake.[155] This influence may be especially important in the context of case-control studies, in which the possibility exists that cases but not controls may alter their diets subsequent to the diagnosis of their disease. Several studies have found a relation between specific food stuffs and Parkinson's disease. These results are, however, still tentative. For example, one study showed that a "protective" effect with peanut consumption was seen only in females, and salad with dressing only in males.[85] Nuts and seeds seemed to be harmful in yet another study.[77] The most impressive data come from a large prospective cohort study of 41 836 women, who have been followed up for six years. In this study there was no association between vitamin E and Parkinson's disease but a significant protective effect was seen for both vitamin C and manganese consumption, whereas vitamin A was associated with an increased risk.[112] The failure of the DATATOP trial to show any benefit with α-tocopherol[156] should not be interpreted as excluding the potential role of dietary antioxidants. Firstly, it is possible that the wrong intervention was chosen, and secondly, dietary factors may protect disease onset (induction) and yet have little effect on prognosis once disease is established (promotion). For example, stopping smoking after the diagnosis of lung cancer has little effect on survival. Given the possible role of antioxidants in the aetiology of Parkinson's disease, these results need confirmation using validated methods of dietary assessment such as seven-day weighed diaries and prospective follow up. In view of the long latency period, it will also be important to consider both adult and childhood diet.

Comment

Various studies have raised the possibility that several different environmental exposures might be related to Parkinson's disease. A toxic exposure is perhaps the most attractive suggestion as it would be consistent with both the evidence on oxidative damage as well as genetic variations in detoxification systems. Several studies suggest pesticides to be of importance, yet this finding is not consistent and is still relatively non-specific. It is important that we collect more data on this exposure and refine current methods of exposure measurement, by combining self reporting measures with biological variables. Prospective occupational cohort studies among those known to have high exposures will need to confirm these associations and identify whether any risk is linked to a specific agent or a broader class of exposures. Infectious exposures seem, if anything, to be less frequent in cases of Parkinson's disease. The interpretation of this finding is uncertain and further work is required to examine not only exposure, but also age at exposure. Self recall data will be problematic and other proxy markers, such as household size, measures of crowding, etc should also be examined. The inverse relation between smoking and Parkinson's disease remains enigmatic but deserves further attention, particularly in relation to premorbid personality differences. In the future, cohort studies

23

with data on personality and behaviour of children will eventually have sufficient cases of Parkinson's disease to test these questions definitively. At the moment these cohorts are still relatively young and have too few patients with Parkinson's disease. Head trauma cannot be definitively excluded as a risk factor, despite a negative cohort study of subjects with past head injury. Larger cohorts with documented injury or occupational cohorts at high risk of head trauma should be examined. Laboratory work is also needed to examine the biological plausibility of minor trauma precipitating a chain of biochemical events that result in cell death. The association between rural residence, well water consumption, and Parkinson's disease initially seemed to be a consistent and potentially important clue. However, the absence of any association in a population based case-control study is a serious concern as prior results may have been influenced by selection bias. This finding needs confirmation by further suitable studies. Population based prevalence studies comparing stable urban and rural populations in the same country will definitively answer whether there is any excess risk associated with residence in a rural area. The role of dietary factors is still unclear as current evidence is weak. More complex methods of dietary measurement using prospective cohorts would establish whether these results are artefactual.

Comorbidity

The association between Parkinson's disease and other diseases can be a useful clue as to shared common aetiological factors, be they genetic or environmental.

Cardiovascular disease, hypertension, and diabetes

Heart disease and stroke have been reported to be less common in male patients with Parkinson's disease[72] or to be no different from the general population.[157] Most studies which have reported causes of death for patients with Parkinson's disease have used proportional mortality[50 158 159] and have therefore potentially underestimated the relevance of heart disease compared with the general population.[71] One cohort study has reported a twofold to threefold increased risk for both heart disease and stroke compared with normal controls.[49] However, this has not been

24

replicated.[52] Hypertension has either been less common[99 157] or no different from control groups.[72 79 80] This might relate to abnormalities in autonomic control mechanisms. No increased risk has been seen for diabetes[79 80 160] despite the experimental finding that fructose blocks MPTP toxicity in isolated hepatocytes.[161]

Malignancy

Several studies have shown that patients with Parkinson's disease experience about half the number of cancers than would be expected from general population rates.[49 159 162–164] When this is examined in more detail, this deficit is specifically related to smoking related cancers[49 162] and is simply explained by the larger proportion of never smokers in the Parkinson's disease population.

Comment

Patients with Parkinson's disease have a different comorbidity profile than normal controls. The risk of cancers is lower as smoking related malignancies are less common. This is simply explained by the lower prevalence rates of smoking. It is unclear whether the risk of cardiovascular disease is increased in patients with Parkinson's disease.

Conclusions

There is little doubt that Parkinson's disease and other neurodegenerative diseases will increase in importance over the next few decades as the population continues to age and many of the other important causes of morbidity continue to decline.[165] Epidemiological research on Parkinson's disease has flourished over the past 10 years, but many findings are still tentative or inconsistent. Future descriptive studies should focus on populations with either anomalous high or low rates of Parkinson's disease. High quality temporal data are essential to determine whether incidence rates are heterogenous depending on age and sex. Better data on elderly cohorts will clarify whether incidence of Parkinson's disease increases exponentially with age. Specific exposures need to be tested more rigorously, either by using special "at risk" cohorts, or by improving measurement of exposure, such as prospective cohorts with reliable measures of dietary intake. Our growing understanding of both the basic pathology and the possible role of genetic factors suggests that certain subgroups of the population may be more susceptible to potential environmental factors. Epidemiologists will need to collaborate with laboratory based researchers to disentangle the relative importance of each risk factor and examine for potential interactions.

I thank the two anonymous referees for useful comments on the initial version of this paper. Much of my knowledge about the epidemiology of Parkinson's disease was acquired while funded by a Wellcome Trust fellowship in clinical epidemiology.

1 Parkinson J. *An essay on the shaking palsy*. London: Sherwood, Neely, and Jones, 1817:1–66
2 Koller WC, Wong GF, Lang A. Posttraumatic movement disorders: a review. *Mov Disord* 1989;4:20–36.
3 Factor SA, Sanchez Ramos J, Weiner WJ. Trauma as an etiology of parkinsonism: a historical review of the concept. *Mov Disord* 1988;3:30–6.
4 Stern MB. Head trauma as a risk factor for Parkinson's disease. *Mov Disord* 1991;6:95–7.
5 Khoury MJ, Beaty TH, Cohen BH. *Fundamentals of genetic epidemiology*. New York: Oxford University Press, 1993:3–383
6 Sasco AJ, Paffenbarger RS. Measles infection and Parkinson's disease. *Am J Epidemiol* 1985;122:1017–31.
7 Ben-Shlomo Y, Sieradzan K. Idiopathic parkinson's disease: epidemiology, diagnosis and management. *Br J Gen Pract* 1995;45:261–8.
8 Mutch WJ, Dingwall-Fordyce I, Downie AW, Paterson JG, Roy SK. Parkinson's disease in a Scottish city. *BMJ* 1986;292:534–6.
9 Harada H, Nishikawa S, Takahashi K. Epidemiology of Parkinson's disease in a Japanese city. *Arch Neurol* 1983;40:151–4.
10 Martilla RJ, Rinne UK. Epidemiology of Parkinson's disease in Finland. *Acta Neurol Scand* 1976;53:81–102.
11 Hughes AJ, Daniel SE, Kilford L, Lees AJ. Accuracy of clinical diagnosis of idiopathic Parkinson's disease: a clinico-pathological study of 100 cases. *J Neurol Neurosurg Psychiatry* 1992;55:181–4.
12 Hughes AJ, Ben-Shlomo Y, Daniel SE, Lees AJ. What features improve the accuracy of clinical diagnosis in Parkinson's disease: a clinicopathological study. *Neurology* 1992;42:1142–6.
13 Riggs JE. Smoking and Alzheimer's disease: protective effect or differential survival bias? *Lancet* 1993;342:793–4.
14 Mattock C, Marmot M, Stern G. Could Parkinson's disease follow intra-uterine influenza?: a speculative hypothesis. *J Neurol Neurosurg Psychiatry* 1988;51:753–6.
15 Eldridge R, Ince SE. The low concordance rate for Parkinson's disease in twins: a possible explanation. *Neurology* 1984;34:1354–6.
16 Calne DB, Langston JW. Aetiology of Parkinson's disease. *Lancet* 1983;2:1457–9.
17 Langston JW. Predicting Parkinson's disease. *Neurology* 1990;40:70–4.
18 Koller WC, Langston JW, Hubble JP, *et al*. Does a long preclinical period occur in Parkinson's disease?. *Neurology* 1991;41:8–13.

19 Koller WC. When does Parkinson's disease begin? *Neurology* 1992;**42** (suppl 4):27–31.

20 Gibb WR, Lees AJ. The progression of idiopathic Parkinson's disease is not explained by age-related changes. Clinical and pathological comparisons with post-encephalitic parkinsonian syndrome. *Acta Neuropathol (Berl)* 1987;**73**:195–201.

21 Schulzer M, Lee CS, Mak EK, Vingerhoets JG, Calne DB. A mathematical model of pathogenesis in idiopathic parkinsonism. *Brain* 1994;**117**:509–16.

22 Goldberg ID, Kurland LT. Mortality in 33 countries from diseases of the nervous system. *World Neurology* 1962;**3**:444–63.

23 Williams GR. Morbidity and mortality with parkinsonism. *J Neurosurg* 1966;**24** (suppl):138–43.

24 Zhang Z, Roman GC. Worldwide occurence of Parkinson's disease: an updated review. *Neuroepidemiology* 1993;**12**:195–208.

25 Hayward RA, Shapiro MF, Freeman HE, Corey CR. Inequities in health services among insured Americans. *N Engl J Med* 1988;**318**:1507–12.

26 Schoenberg BS, Anderson DW, Haerer AF. Prevalence of Parkinson's disease in the biracial population of Copiah County, Mississippi. *Neurology* 1985;**35**:841–5.

27 de Pedro-Cuesta J. *Parkinson's disease diagnostic criteria, incidence and etiology: III Europarkinson Workshop.* Madrid: Institute of Health, 1991.

28 Wang SJ, Fuh JL, Liu CY, *et al.* Parkinson's disease in Kin-Hu, Kinmen: a community survey by neurologists. *Neuroepidemiology* 1994;**13**:69–74.

29 Jendroska K, Olasode BJ, Daniel SE, *et al.* Incidental Lewy body disease in black Africans. *Lancet* 1994;**344**:882–3.

30 Ben-Shlomo Y, Wenning G. Incidental Lewy body disease. *Lancet* 1994;**344**:1503.

31 Tanner CM, Chen B, Wang W, *et al.* Environmental factors and Parkinson's disease: a case-control study in China. *Neurology* 1989;**39**:660–4.

32 Marmot MG, Adelstein AM, Bulusu L. Lessons from the study of immigrant mortality. *Lancet* 1984;**i**:1455–8.

33 Gudmundsson KR. A clinical survey of Parkinsonism in Iceland. *Acta Neurol Scand* 1967;**43** (suppl 33):9–61.

34 de Pedro-Cuesta J, Petersen IJ, Stawiarz L, *et al.* High levodopa use in periodically time-clustered, Icelandic birth cohorts. A vestige of parkinsonism etiology? *Acta Neurol Scand* 1995;**91**:79–88.

35 Manyam BV. Paralysis agitans and levodopa in "Ayurveda": ancient Indian medical treatise. *Mov Disord* 1990;**5**:47–8.

36 Kurtzke JF, Murphy FM. The changing patterns of death rates in parkinsonism. *Neurology* 1990;**40**:42–9.

37 Treves TA, de Pedro-Cuesta J. Parkinsonism mortality in the US, 1. Time and space distribution. *Acta Neurol Scand* 1991;**84**:389–97.

38 Lilienfeld DE, Chan E, Ehland J, *et al.* Two decades of increasing mortality from Parkinson's disease among the US elderly. *Arch Neurol* 1990;**47**:731–4.

39 Duvoisin RC, Schweitzer MD. Paralysis agitans mortality in England and Wales, 1855–1962. *Br J Prev Soc Med* 1966;**20**:27–33.

40 Marmot MG. Parkinson's disease and encephalitis: the cohort hypothesis re-examined. In: Rose FC, ed. *Clinical Neuroepidemiology.* Kent: Pitman Medical, 1980;391–401.

41 Li T, Swash M, Alberman E. Morbidity and mortality in motor neuron disease: comparison with multiple sclerosis and Parkinson's disease: age and sex specific rates and cohort analyses. *J Neurol Neurosurg Psychiatry* 1985;**48**:320–7.

42 Clarke CE. Mortality from Parkinson's disease in England and Wales 1921–1989. *J Neurol Neurosurg Psychiatry* 1993;**56**:690–3.

43 Ben-Shlomo Y, Finnan F, Allwright S, Davey Smith G. The epidemiology of Parkinson's disease in Ireland: observations from routine data sources. *Ir Med J* 1993;**86**:190–4.

44 Vanacore N, Bonifati V, Bellatreccia A, Edito F, Meco G. Mortality rates for Parkinson's disease and parkinsonism in Italy (1969–1987). *Neuroepidemiology* 1992;**11**:65–73.

45 Kurtzke JF, Flaten TP, Murphy FM. Death rates from Parkinson's disease in Norway reflect increased survival. *Neurology* 1991;**41**:1665–7.

46 Imaizumi Y, Kaneko R. Rising mortality from Parkinson's disease in Japan, 1950–1992. *Acta Neurol Scand* 1995;**91**:169–76.

47 Clarke CE. Does levodopa therapy delay death in Parkinson's disease? A review of the evidence. *Mov Disord* 1995;**10**:250–6.

48 Ebmeier KP, Calder SA, Crawford JR, Stewart L, Beeson JAO, Mutch WJ. Parkinson's disease in Aberdeen: survival after 3·5 years. *Acta Neurol Scand* 1990;**81**:294–9.

49 Ben-Shlomo Y, Marmot MG. Survival and cause of death in a cohort of patients with parkinsonism: possible clues to aetiology. *J Neurol Neurosurg Psychiatry* 1995;**58**:293–9.

50 Hoehn MM, Yahr MD. Parkinsonism: onset, progression, and mortality. *Neurology* 1967;**17**:427–42.

51 Riggs JE, Schochet SS. Rising mortality due to Parkinson's disease and amyotrophic lateral sclerosis: a manifestation of the competitive nature of human mortality. *J Clin Epidemiol* 1992;**45**:1007–12.

52 Bennett DA, Beckett LA, Murray AM, *et al.* Prevalence of Parkinsonian signs and associated mortality in a community population of older people. *N Engl J Med* 1996;**334**:71–6.

53 Poskanzer DC, Schwab RS. Cohort analysis of Parkinson's syndrome. Evidence for a single etiology related to subclinical infection about 1920. *J Chron Dis* 1963;**16**:961–73.

54 Brown EL, Knox EG. Epidemiological approach to Parkinson's disease. *Lancet* 1972;**1**:974–6.

55 Holford TR. Analysing the temporal effects of age, period and cohort. *Statistical Methods in Medical Research* 1992;**1**:317–37.

56 Ravenholt RT, Foege WH. 1918 Influenza, encephalitis lethargica, parkinsonism. *Lancet* 1982;**ii**:860–4.

57 Kurland LT, Hauser WA, Okazaki H, Nobrega FT. Epidemiologic studies of Parkinsonism with special reference to the cohort hypothesis. In: *Proceedings of the third symposium on Parkinsonism.* Edinburgh: Livingstone, 1969:12–6.

58 Nobrega FT, Glattre E, Kurland LT, Okazaki H. Comments on the epidemiology of parkinsonism including prevalence and incidence statistics for Rochester, Minnesota, 1953–1966. In: Barbeau A, Brunette JR, eds. *Progress in Neurogenetics.* Amsterdam: Excerpta Medica, 1969:474–85.

59 Rajput AH, Offord KP, Beard CM, Kurland LT. Epidemiology of parkinsonism: incidence, classification and mortality. *Ann Neurol* 1984;**16**:278–82.

60 de Pedro-Cuesta J, Stawiarz L. Parkinson's disease incidence: magnitude, comparability, time trends. *Acta Neurol Scand* 1991;**84**:382–8.

61 Ritchie K, Kildea D. Is senile dementia "age-related" or ageing-related"?— evidence from meta-analysis of dementia prevalence in the oldest old. *Lancet* 1995;**346**:931–4.

62 Larsen JP and the Norwegian Study Group of Parkinson's disease in the elderly. Parkinson's disease as community health problem: study in Norwegian nursing homes. *BMJ* 1991;**303**:741–3.

63 Li S, Schoenberg BS, Wang C, *et al.* A prevalence survey of Parkinson's disease and other movement disorders in the People's Republic of China. *Arch Neurol* 1985;**42**:655–7.

64 Morgante L, Rocca WA, Di Rosa AE, et al. Prevalence of Parkinson's disease and other types of parkinsonism: a door-to-door survey in three Sicillian municipalities. Neurology 1992;42:1901–7.

65 Bharucha NE, Bharucha EP, Bharucha AE, Bhise AV, Schoenberg BS. Prevalence of Parkinson's disease in the Parsi community of Bombay, India. Arch Neurol 1988;45:1321–3.

66 Tison F, Dartigues JF, Dubes L, Zuber M, Alperovitch A, Henry P. Prevalence of Parkinson's disease in the elderly: a population study in Gironde, France. Acta Neurol Scand 1994;90:111–5.

67 Liberatos P, Link BG, Kelsey JL. The measurement of social class in epidemiology. Epidemiol Rev 1988;10:87–121.

68 Marmot MG, Shipley MJ, Rose G. Inequalities in death—specific explanations of a general pattern? Lancet 1984;i:1003–6.

69 Office of Population Census and Surveys. Classification of occupations. London: HMSO, 1980

70 McKeigue PM, Marmot MG. Epidemiology of Parkinson's disease. In: Stern G, ed. Parkinson's disease. London: Chapman and Hall, 1989:295–306.

71 Breslow NE, Day NE. Statistical methods in cancer research: Volume 2—the design and analysis of cohort studies. Lyon: IARC:1987.

72 Kessler II. Epidemiologic studies of Parkinson's disease. III. A community based survey. Am J Epidemiol 1972;96:242–54.

73 Martilla RJ, Rinne UK. Arteriosclerosis, hereditary and some previous infections in the aetiology of Parkinson's disease. A case control study. Clin Neurol Neurosurg 1976;79:46–56.

74 Stern M, Dulaney E, Gruber SB, et al. The epidemiology of Parkinson's disease: a case-control study of young-onset and old-onset patients. Arch Neurol 1991;48:903–7.

75 Semchuck KM, Love EJ, Lee RG. Parkinson's disease and exposure to agricultural work and pesticide chemicals. Neurology 1992;42:1328–35.

76 Mayeux R, Tang MX, Marder K, Cote LJ, Stern Y. Smoking and Parkinson's disease. Mov Disord 1994;9:207–12.

77 Butterfield PG, Valanis BG, Spencer PS, Lindeman CA, Nutt JG. Environmental antecedents of young-onset Parkinson's disease. Neurology 1993;43:1150–8.

78 Bharucha NE, Stokes L, Schoenberg BS, et al. A case-control study of twin pairs discordant for Parkinson's disease: a search for environmental risk factors. Neurology 1986;36:284–8.

79 Grandinetti A, Morens DM, Reed D, MacEachern D. Prospective study of cigarette smoking and the risk of developing idiopathic Parkinson's disease. Am J Epidemiol 1994;139:1129–38.

80 Ho SC, Woo J, Lee CM. Epidemiologic study of Parkinson's disease in Hong Kong. Neurology 1989;39:1314–8.

81 Hubble JP, Cao T, Hassanein RE, Neuberger JS, Koller WC. Risk factors for Parkinson's disease. Neurology 1993;43:1693–7.

82 Wong GF, Gray CS, Hassanein RS, Koller WC. Environmental risk factors in siblings with Parkinson's disease. Arch Neurol 1991;48:287–9.

83 Koller W, Vetere-Overfield B, Gray C, et al. Environmental risk factors in Parkinson's disease. Neurology 1990;40:1218–21.

84 Barbeau A, Roy M, Bernier G, Campanella G, Paris S. Ecogenetics of Parkinson's disease: prevalence and environmental aspects in rural areas. Can J Neurol Sci 1987;14:36–41.

85 Golbe LI, Farrell TM, Davis PH. Follow-up study of early-life protective and risk factors in Parkinson's disease. Mov Disord 1990;5:66–70.

86 Ohlson C, Hogstedt C. Parkinson's disease and occupational exposure to organic solvents, agricultural chemicals and mercury—a case-referent study. Scand J Work Environ Health 1981;7:252–6.

87 Jimenez-Jimenez FJ, Mateo D, Gimenez-Roldan S. Exposure to well water and pesticides in Parkinson's disease: a case-control study in the Madrid area. *Mov Disord* 1992;7:149–52.

88 Ngim C, Devathasan G. Epidemiologic study on the association between body burden mercury level and idiopathic Parkinson's disease. *Neuroepidemiology* 1989;8:128–41.

89 Aquilonius SM, Hartvig P. A Swedish county with unexpectedly high utilization of anti-parkinsonian drugs. *Acta Neurol Scand* 1986;74:379–82.

90 Wang WZ, Fang XH, Cheng XM, Jiang DH, Lin ZJ. A case-control study on the environmental risk factors of Parkinson's disease in Tianjin, China. *Neuroepidemiology* 1993;12:209–18.

91 Ebmeier KP, Mutch WJ, Calder SA, Crawford JR, Stewart L, Besson JO. Does idiopathic Parkinsonism in Aberdeen follow intrauterine influenza? *J Neurol Neurosurg Psychiatry* 1989;52:911–3.

92 Baumann RJ, Jameson HD, McKean HE, Haack DG, Weisberg LM. Cigarette smoking and Parkinson disease: 1. A comparison of cases with matched neighbours. *Neurology* 1980;30:839–43.

93 Godwin-Austen RB, Lee PN, Marmot MG, Stern GM. Smoking and Parkinson's disease. *J Neurol Neurosurg Psychiatry* 1982;45:577–81.

94 Kondo K. Epidemiological evaluations of risk factors in Parkinson's disease. *Adv Neurol* 1987;45:289–93.

95 Semchuk KM, Love EJ, Lee RG. Parkinson's disease: a test of the multifactorial etiologic hypothesis. *Neurology* 1993;43:1173–80.

96 Nefzger MD, Quadfasel FA, Karl VC. A retrospective study of smoking in Parkinson's disease. *Am J Epidemiol* 1968;88:149–58.

97 Martilla RJ, Rinne UK. Smoking and Parkinson's disease. *Acta Neurol Scand* 1980;62:322–25.

98 Haack DG, Baumann RJ, McKean HE, Jameson HD, Turbek JA. Nicotine exposure and Parkinson disease. *Am J Epidemiol* 1981;114:191–9.

99 Rajput AH, Offord KP, Beard CM, Kurland LT. A case-control study of smoking habits, dementia, and other illnesses in idiopathic Parkinson's disease. *Neurology* 1987;37:226–32.

100 Jimenez Jimenez FJ, Mateo D, Gimenez Roldan S. Premorbid smoking, alcohol consumption, and coffee drinking habits in Parkinson's disease: a case-control study. *Mov Disord* 1992;7:339–44.

101 Kahn HA. The Dorn study of smoking and mortality among U.S. Veterans: report on eight and one-half years of observation. *Nat Cancer Inst Monogr* 1966;19:1–125.

102 Hammond EC. Smoking in relation to the death rates of one million men and women. In: Haenzel W, ed. *Epidemiological approaches to the study of cancer and other chronic diseases.* Bethesda, MD: National Cancer Institute, 1966:127–204. *(National Cancer Institute Monograph No 19.)*

103 Doll R, Peto R, Wheatley K, Gray R, Sutherland I. Mortality in relation to smoking: 40 years' observations on male British doctors. *BMJ* 1994;309:901–11.

104 Sasco AJ, Paffenbarger RSJ. Smoking and Parkinson's disease. *Epidemiology* 1990;1:460–5.

105 Poewe W, Karamat E, Kemmler GW, Gerstenbrand F. The premorbid personality of patients with Parkinson's disease: a comparative study with healthy controls and patients with essential tremor. *Adv Neurol* 1990;53:339–42.

106 Eatough VM, Kempster PA, Stern GM, Lees AJ. Premorbid personality and idiopathic Parkinson's disease. *Adv Neurol* 1990;53:335–7.

107 Ward CD, Duvoisin RC, Ince SE, Nutt JD, Eldridge R, Calne DB. Parkinson's disease in 65 pairs of twins and in a set of quadruplets. *Neurology* 1983;33:815–24.

108 Williams DB, Annegers JF, Kokmen E, O'Brien PC, Kurland LT. Brain injury and neurologic sequelae: a cohort study of dementia, parkinsonism, and amyotrophic lateral sclerosis. *Neurology* 1991;**41**:1554–7.
109 Semchuck KM, Love EJ, Lee RG. Parkinson's disease and exposure to rural environmental factors: a population based case-control study. *Can J Neurol Sci* 1991;**18**:279–86.
110 Golbe LI, Farrell TM, Davis PH. Case-control study of early life dietary factors in Parkinson's disease. *Arch Neurol* 1988;**45**:1350–3.
111 Tanner CM, Chen B, Cohen JA, et al. Dietary antioxidant vitamins and the risk of developing Parkinson's disease. *Neurology* 1989;**39**:181
112 Cerhan JR, Wallace RB, Folsom AR. Antioxidant intake and risk of Parkinson's disease (PD) in older women. *Am J Epidemiol* 1994;**139**:S65.
113 Lang AE, Marsden CD, Obeso JA, Parkes JD. Alcohol and Parkinson disease. *Ann Neurol* 1982;**12**:254–6.
114 Langston JW, Ballard P, Tetrud JW, Irwin I. Chronic parkinsonism in humans due to a product of meperidine-analog synthesis. *Science* 1983;**219**:970–80.
115 Tanner CM, Langston JW. Do environmental toxins cause Parkinson's disease? A critical review. *Neurology* 1990;**40**:suppl 30.
116 Sanchez-Ramos JR, Hefti F, Weiner WJ. Paraquat and Parkinson's disease. *Neurology* 1987;**37**:728.
117 Blair A, Zahm SH. Patterns of pesticide use among farmers: implications for epidemiologic research. *Epidemiology* 1993;**4**:55–62.
118 Stephens R, Spurgeon A, Calvert IA, et al. Neuropsychological effects of long-term exposure to organophosphates in sheep dip. *Lancet* 1995;**345**:1135–9.
119 Robins AH. Depression in patients with parkinsonism. *Br J Psychiatry* 1976;**128**:141–5.
120 Cummings JL. Depression and Parkinson's disease: a review. *Am J Psychiatry* 1992;**149**:443–54.
121 Yesalis CEI, Lemke JH, Wallace RB, Kohonut FJ, Morris MC. Health status of the rural elderly according to farm work history: the Iowa 65+ rural health study. *Arch Environ Health* 1985;**40**:245–50.
122 Tanner C. Abnormal liver enzyme-mediated metabolism in Parkinson's disease: a second look. *Neurology* 1991;**41**:89–91.
123 Steventon GB, Heafield MTE, Waring RH, Williams AC. Xenobiotic metabolism in Parkinson's disease. *Neurology* 1989;**39**:883–7.
124 Steventon GB, Heafield MTE, Sturman SG, Waring RH, Williams AC, Ellingham J. Degenerative neurological disease and debrisoquine-4-hydroxylation capacity. *Medical Science Research* 1989;**17**:163–4.
125 Armstrong M, Daly AK, Cholerton S, Bateman DN, Idle JR. Mutant debrisoquine hydroxylation genes in Parkinson's disease. *Lancet* 1992;**339**:1017–8.
126 Smith CAD, Gough AC, Leigh PN, et al. Debrisoquine hydroxylase gene polymorphism and suceptibility to Parkinson's disease. *Lancet* 1992; **339**:1375–7.
127 Agid Y. Parkinson's disease: pathophysiology. *Lancet* 1991;**337**:1321–3.
128 Elizan TS, Madden DL, Noble GR, et al. Viral antibodies in serum and CSF of parkinsonian patients and controls. *Arch Neurol* 1979;**36**:529–34.
129 Martilla RJ, Arstila P, Nikostelainen J, Halonen PE, Rinne UK. Viral antibodies in the sera from patients with Parkinson's disease. *Eur Neurol* 1977;**15**:25–33.
130 Schwartz J, Elizan TS. Search for viral particles and virus-specific products in idiopathic Parkinson disease brain material. *Ann Neurol* 1979;**6**:261–3.
131 Martyn CN, Cruddas M, Compston DA. Symptomatic Epstein-Barr virus infection and multiple sclerosis. *J Neurol Neurosurg Psychiatry* 1993;**56**:167–8.

31

132 Riggs JE. Cigarette smoking and Parkinson disease: the illusion of a neuroprotective effect. *Clin Neuropharmacol* 1992;**15**:88–99.

133 Ben-Shlomo Y. Smoking and neurodegenerative diseases. *Lancet* 1993;**342**:1239.

134 Yong VW, Perry TL. Monoamine oxidase B, smoking and Parkinson's disease. *J Neurol Sci* 1986;**72**:265–72.

135 Jenner P. Oxidative damage in neurodegenerative disease. *Lancet* 1994; **344**:796–8.

136 Smith PR, Cooper JM, Govan GG, Harding AE, Schapira AHV. Smoking and mitochondrial function: a model for environmental toxins. *Q J Med* 1993;**86**:657–60.

137 Gresham LS, Molgaard CA, Smith RA. Induction of cytochrome P-450 enzymes via tobacco smoke: a potential mechanism for developing resistance to environmental toxins as related to parkinsonism and other neurologic diseases. *Neuroepidemiology* 1993;**12**:114–6.

138 Golbe LI, Cody RA, Duvoisin RC. Smoking and Parkinson's disease: search for a dose-response relationship. *Arch Neurol* 1986;**43**:774–80.

139 Eysenck HJ, Tarrant M, Woolf M, England L. Smoking and personality. *BMJ* 1960;**i**:456–60.

140 Forgays DG, Bonaiuto P, Wrzesniewski K, Forgays DK. Personality and cigarette smoking in Italy, Poland and the United States. *Int J Addict* 1993;**28**:399–413.

141 Plassman BL, Helms MJ, Welsh KA, Saunders AM, Breitner JCS. Smoking, Alzheimer' disease and confounding with genes. *Lancet* 1995;**345**:387.

142 Godwin Austen RB, Lee PN, Marmot MG, Stern GM. Smoking and Parkinson's disease. *J Neurol Neurosurg Psychiatry* 1982;**45**:577–81.

143 Raphael K. Recall bias: a proposal for assessment and control. *Int J Epidemiol* 1987;**16**:167–70.

144 Weiss N. Should we consider a subject's knowledge of the etiologic hypothesis in the analysis of case-control studies? *Am J Epidemiol* 1994;**139**:247–9.

145 Rajput AH, Utti RJ, Stern W, Laverty W. Early onset Parkinson's disease in Saskatchewan—environmental considerations for etiology. *Can J Neurol Sci* 1986;**13**:312–6.

146 Martyn CN. Choosing cases and controls in neurological research. *J Neurol Neurosurg Psychiatry* 1990;**53**:453–4.

147 Blazer DG, Landerman LR, Fillenbaum G, Horner R. Health services access and use among older adults in North Carolina: urban vs rural residents. *Am J Public Health* 1995;**85**:1384–90.

148 Rybicki BA, Johnson CC, Gorell JM. Demographic differences in referral rates to neurologists of patients with suspected Parkinson's disease: implications for case-control study design. *Neuroepidemiology* 1995;**14**:72–81.

149 Schlesselman JJ. *Case-control studies: design, conduct, analysis*. New York: Oxford University Press, 1982:1–354.

150 Granieri E, Carreras M, Casetta I, *et al.* Parkinson's disease in Ferrara, Italy, 1967 through 1987. *Arch Neurol* 1991;**49**:854–7.

151 Phillips AN, Davey Smith G. How independent are "independent" effects? Relative risk estimation when correlated exposures are measured imprecisely. *J Clin Epidemiol* 1991;**44**:1223–31.

152 Rajput AH, Uitti RJ, Stern W, *et al.* Geography, drinking water chemistry, pesticides and herbicides and the etiology of Parkinson's disease. *Can J Neurol Sci* 1987;**14**:414–8.

153 Spencer P. Guam ALS/Parkinsonism-dementia: a long-latency neurotoxic disorder caused by "slow toxin(s)" in food? *Can J Neurol Sci* 1987;**14**:347–57.

154 Willett W. Overview of nutritional epidemiology. In: Willett W, ed. *Nutritional epidemiology*. New York: Oxford University Press, 1990;3–19.

155 Dwyer JT, Gardner J, Halvorsen K, Krall EA, Cohen A, Valadian I. Memory of food intake in the distant past. *Am J Epidemiol* 1989;**130**:1033–46.

156 The Parkinson Study Group. Effects of tocopherol and deprenyl on the progression of disability in early Parkinson's disease. *N Engl J Med* 1993; **328**:176–83.

157 Marttila RJ, Rinne UK. Arteriosclerosis, heredity, and some previous infections in the etiology of Parkinson's disease. A case-control study. *Clin Neurol Neurosurg* 1976;**79**:46–56.

158 Hoehn MMM. Parkinson's disease: progression and mortality. *Adv Neurol* 1986;**45**:457–61.

159 Marmot MG. Mortality and Parkinson's disease. In: Rose FC, Capildeo R, eds. *Research progress in Parkinson's disease*. London: Pitman, 1988;9–16.

160 Rajput AH, Offord KP, Beard CM, Kurland LT. A case-control study of smoking habits, dementia, and other illnesses in idiopathic Parkinson's disease. *Neurology* 1987;**37**:226–32.

161 Di Monte D, Sandy MS, Blank L, Smith MT. Fructose prevents 1-methyl-4-phenyl-1,2,3,6-tetrahydropyridine (MPTP)-induced ATP depletion and toxicity in isolated hepatocytes. *Biochem Biophys Res Commun* 1988; **153**:734–40.

162 Moller H, Mellemkjaer L, McLaughlin JK, Olsen JH. Occurence of different cancers in patients with Parkinson's disease. *BMJ* 1995;**310**:1500–1.

163 Barbeau A, Joly JG. Parkinson et cancer. *Union Med Can* 1963;**92**:169–74.

164 Jansson B, Jankovic J. Low cancer rates among patients with Parkinson's disease. *Ann Neurol* 1985;**17**:505–9.

165 Barrett-Connor E. Are we living longer or dying longer? In: Poulter N, Sever P, Thom S, eds. *Cardiovascular disease: risk factors and intervention*. Oxford: Radcliffe Medical Press, 1993:89–99.

2 Schizophrenia

MARY CANNON, PETER JONES

> - There is evidence that rates of schizophrenia are higher in developing countries than in the developed world.
> - Incidence rates seem to be declining in many developed countries.
> - The onset of schizophrenia tends to occur in late adolescence or early adult life. This is unusual for chronic diseases. Age at onset tends to be 3–4 years earlier in men than women.
> - Impairments in motor and cognitive development are frequently present in children long before the onset of psychotic symptoms.
> - Schizophrenia has strong genetic determinants but risk factors operating pre-natally and perinatally are also important.
> - Schizophrenia may be a neurodevelopmental disorder.

Psychiatric epidemiology is the study of the distribution and causes of mental disorder in the population. Over the past 30 years progress in psychiatric epidemiology has been slower than in other areas—for example, cardiovascular disease or cancer epidemiology, because of certain methodological problems that are just now being overcome. In particular the epidemiology of schizophrenia has suffered from two major difficulties: uncertainty about how to define a case, and the relative rarity of schizophrenia in the population.

Special methodological problems in schizophrenia epidemiology

What is a case

The lack of physical signs or laboratory tests means that a diagnosis of schizophrenia is based on evaluation of patients' self reported, subjective experiences. Until the late 1960s, there was a relatively loose definition of schizophrenia and a good deal of diagnostic latitude was allowed to individual psychiatrists. However, a report published in 1972,[1] showed that the diagnostic habits of psychiatrists in the United States and United Kingdom differed to an unacceptable degree, and led to the introduction of strict operational diagnostic criteria for schizophrenia. The Diagnostic and Statistical Manual DSM-III,[2] published in 1980, reduced the reliance on symptoms alone by incorporating an element of chronicity—six months prior duration of symptoms and an upper age limit of 45 years for a first diagnosis of schizophrenia. Since 1980 there have been two more restrictive revisions of this diagnostic system, DSM-III-R[3] and DSM-IV,[4] and the International Classification of Diseases, (ICD), the diagnostic system favoured by European psychiatrists, has also undergone a similar "narrowing" process with the change from ICD-9 to ICD-10.[5]

But has this process gone too far? Although the restrictive diagnostic criteria have certainly increased the *reliability* of the diagnosis, they have not improved the *validity* of "DSM-IV" or "ICD-10 schizophrenia".[6] Recent family studies indicate that a broader concept of schizophrenia actually fits genetic models more readily than a restrictive definition. In addition, the frequent changes in diagnostic criteria have affected the comparability of studies of time trends and outcome in schizophrenia. Also, the commitment to a phenotype based on symptoms in adult life may have ignored an important developmental or lifelong dimension to the disorder.

Schizophrenia as a "rare disease"

The low incidence (10–40 cases per 100 000 per year) and relatively low lifetime prevalence (0·5%–1%) of schizophrenia in the population have led to a reliance on case-control study designs in research. Chronic patients recruited from hospital wards are compared with volunteer controls from the community and consequent problems of bias and confounding have often led to unreplicated and contradictory findings. It seemed for a time that schizophrenia, already known as the "graveyard of neuropathologists",[7] would also prove to be the undoing of epidemiologists. Over the past two decades, however, the application of advances in case-control methodology to psychiatric epidemiology has led to more robust results.[8] Also, cohort designs, for long thought too costly and time consuming to use in schizophrenia research, have made a "comeback".

For the purposes of this review schizophrenia refers to a recent, operational definition such as CATEGO,[9] ICD-10, DSM-III, DSM-III-R, or DSM-IV. Robust findings are those from studies with an epidemiological design— that is, population based studies with well defined samples and appropriate controls. We aim to show how the findings from robust epidemiological research can help to unravel the complex aetiology of schizophrenia.

Geography

In 1978, a large multicentre study of schizophrenia was initiated by WHO—the 10 country study (also known as the Determinants of Outcome of Severe Mental Disorders Study), to provide information about the incidence, course, and outcome of schizophrenia in different cultures.[10] Two case definitions of schizophrenia were used: a broad, clinical definition comprising ICD-9 schizophrenia and paranoid psychoses, and a narrow, restrictive definition including only cases classified as "nuclear" schizophrenia using the CATEGO computer programme.[9] Figures 2.1a and b show the incidence rates for both definitions. There is little variation between centres for narrowly defined schizophrenia with rates ranging only between 7 and 14/100 000, (fig 2.1a). Although the parsimonious conclusion would be that the rates for narrowly defined schizophrenia are the same, the confidence intervals for these estimates were wide and there may not have been sufficient statistical power to detect differences.

The incidence rates for broadly defined schizophrenia do seem to vary between countries (range 16 to 42/100 000 per year), and the rates for centres in the developing world are about twice as high as those in the developed world (fig 2.1b). Further studies of schizophrenia in the developing world are needed to replicate and further investigate these interesting findings, and the problem of mental health in the developing world can no longer remain a low priority for funding agencies and governments. On the whole, however, the variation in incidence rates for schizophrenia world wide is very small compared with illnesses such as ischaemic heart disease or cancer, which are known to have major environmental risk factors.

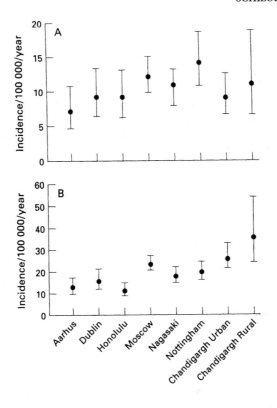

Figure 2.1   (a) Incidence of CATEGO S narrow schizophrenia with 95% confidence intervals from eight centres in the WHO Determinants of Outcome Study. (b) Incidence of CATEGO S, P, and O broad schizophrenia with 95% confidence limits from eight centres in the WHO determinants of outcome study. Data from Jablensky et. al.[10]

Time trends

Prevalence data

Two major prevalence studies of psychiatric illness have been carried out in the United States, which indicate a decrease in prevalence of schizophrenia over one decade. The Epidemiological Catchment Area (ECA) Study surveyed 17 803 persons between 1980 and 1984 and found a lifetime prevalence of schizophrenia of 1·4%.[11] The National Comorbidity Survey (NCS) interviewed 8098 people between 1990 and 1992 and found that lifetime prevalence for the summary category of non-affective psychosis was 0·7%.[12] This discrepancy may be related to issues of sampling, interview methodology, or actual change over time and remains to be clarified by future reports.

A major prevalence study of psychiatric morbidity carried out in the United Kingdom between April and September 1993,[13] found a prevalence rate of 0·4% for functional psychosis among persons aged 16–64 living in private households. This rate is even lower than that found in the national comorbidity survey but as 37% of those who screened positive for psychosis refused a second diagnostic interview, the true prevalence may be higher.[14] At present, it seems that the lifetime prevalence of schizophrenia in the western world lies somewhere between 0·4% and 1·4%, and may have decreased over the past decade.

"Incidence" data

Prevalence of schizophrenia can be influenced by factors such as change in treatment, change in mortality rate, and changes in the age and sex structure of the population, and therefore, examination of incidence rates may be more informative. Ideally, such studies should be based on community incidence samples but, as this is difficult to achieve, case registers and hospital admission data are commonly used.

Eagles and Whalley[15] first reported a decline in the diagnosis of schizophrenia among first admissions in Scotland between 1969 and 1978. There have since been 14 papers examining this issue in England,[16–20] Scotland,[21–23] Denmark,[24 25] New Zealand,[26] Canada,[27] Ireland,[28] the United States,[29] and the Netherlands.[30] Those based on national statistics have found a large (40%–50%) decline in first admission rates for schizophrenia during the 1970s and the 1980s.[17 18 25 26] Findings based on case register data have been less consistent and indeed, two such studies, from Camberwell[17] and Salford[18] in the United Kingdom, actually found a slight increase in the incidence of schizophrenia during the same period. Others have reported a decrease in first admission rates for schizophrenia among female patients only.[22 28 30]

The major question is whether the decrease noted in first admission rates corresponds to an actual decrease in the incidence of the condition. Many factors influence this apparent "administrative decline" in schizophrenia:

1. The introduction of more restrictive diagnostic criteria for

schizophrenia may cause a shift to diagnoses such as "borderline states"[24] or affective psychosis.[29 30]

2. The move to community care over the past two decades could have affected hospital admission rates.[27]

3. Clinicians have become more reluctant to make a diagnosis of schizophrenia on the first hospital admission,[24] and this could lead to a spurious fall in incidence rates over the last few years of the period under observation. The policies of private health insurance companies regarding schizophrenia may be partly responsible for this effect.[29]

4. Changes in the age, sex, and ethnic structure of the population over the period under study have not been taken into account in most studies. The two areas of the United Kingdom which showed an increased incidence of schizophrenia are both areas with a high proportion of immigrants.[17 18] Unfortunately, schizophrenia has such a low incidence that it may be impossible to disentangle all these effects and reach any firm conclusions regarding changes in incidence in the developed world in recent decades.[31]

Characteristics of patients

Age and sex distribution

Total lifetime risk for schizophrenia seems to be equal in both sexes.[10 32] Schizophrenia can occur at any age,[33-35] but onset is commonly in early adulthood—over 70% of incident cases in the WHO 10 country study were between 15 and 35 years of age.[10] The mean age of onset for male patients is three to four years earlier than for female patients, irrespective of whether onset of schizophrenia is defined as the first sign of mental disorder, the first psychotic symptom, or the first hospital admission.[36-38] The peak age of onset for males is between 15 and 30 whereas females have a slower and more even rate of onset with a peak between the ages of 20 and 35 and a second smaller peak after the age of 45, (fig 2.2).[38] No satisfactory explanation yet exists for this sex difference. A protective effect for female sex hormones has been suggested,[39] but has not been proved empirically. The same pattern occurs across countries indicating that it is not an effect of cultural factors.[10]

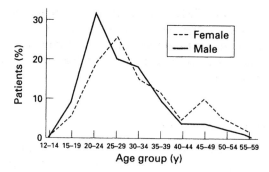

Figure 2.2   Distribution of age at first admission for schizophrenia in males and females. Source: Häfner et al.[38]

Social class

The long recognised association between schizophrenia and low social class was confirmed by the ECA study, which showed that schizophrenic patients in the United States were 10 times more likely to be in the lowest socioeconomic group than in the highest.[35] Evidence from birth cohorts in Britain,[40 41] and Finland[42] show that this relation is not causal—schizophrenic patients at birth have the same socioeconomic distribution as the general population. What is remarkable is the steep decline in social state which accompanies the illness and is evident even before the clinical onset.[42 43] This decline is far greater than that experienced by patients with severe affective disorder.[42 43]

Marital state

Schizophrenic patients have low rates of marriage and low fertility[32]—a challenge to geneticists. Married patients have a better clinical and social outcome than single patients,[10] although marriage may, of course, reflect better premorbid social adjustment and later age at onset, which are both independent predictors of good outcome. However, the prevalence of schizophrenia among separated or divorced people in the United States (2·9%) is similar to that among single people (2·1%), suggesting that marriage may confer an independent protective effect.[32] An interaction between marital state and gender was found in the one year follow up of the ECA study.[44] Single women were 14 times more likely to develop schizophrenia than married women but single men were almost 50 times more likely to develop schizophrenia than their married counterparts. The role of marital state as a risk indicator or modifier for schizophrenia deserves further study.

Ethnicity and migrant state

To date no single *indigenous* ethnic group seems to have a significantly higher rate of schizophrenia than any other,[10] although some pockets of high prevalence may exist in isolated areas like north Sweden.[45] The west of Ireland[46 47] and the Istrian peninsula in Croatia[48] had previously been identified as high risk cultures but the higher rates originally found among these peoples are now thought to be due to methodological factors.[49] Populations with increased prevalence, if carefully identified, could be very useful for geneticists, but they seem to be local exceptions rather than the general rule in the epidemiology of schizophrenia.[50] The ECA study found a higher prevalence for schizophrenia among black people than among white people in the United States (2·1% v 1·4%).[32] However, when controlled for age, gender, marital state, and most importantly, socioeconomic group, the significant difference disappeared. Of course in a cross sectional study such as the ECA study, it is not possible to state definitively that current marital state and socioeconomic state completely explain the association found between race and disorder, because schizophrenia can lead to low social state and marital breakup.

Schizophrenia in immigrants

In 1988, the psychiatric community was surprised by a report that the incidence of schizophrenia among the Afro-Caribbean population in Nottingham was more than 10 times higher than in the general population.[51] This finding has been convincingly replicated in other centres in the United Kingdom[52-55] and in The Netherlands,[56] although the incidence ratio is now thought to be rather lower (3–5) when the denominator is adjusted for possible underreporting in census data.[54 55] An increased incidence ratio for schizophrenia has also been found among African[54 55] and Asian[54] immigrants in the United Kingdom, indicating that the effect is not confined to a single ethnic minority.

41

The hospital admission rate for schizophrenia among migrants is higher in their host country than in their country of origin,[57-59] which implicates factors occurring principally after migration. The risk of schizophrenia is greater among second generation migrants than first generation migrants,[51-54 60] arguing against selective migration of preschizophrenic persons. The fact that immigrants from poor countries tend to show higher rates of schizophrenia than immigrants from affluent countries, implies that factors associated with improved living conditions, industrialisation, or urbanisation are involved. Obstetric complications and exposure to novel viruses during pregnancy have been proposed as biological explanations,[61 62] but empirical evidence is lacking. Two studies have found an increased risk for schizophrenia among the siblings of United Kingdom born Afro-Caribbean schizophrenic patients compared with the risk among siblings of white patients,[63] which could indicate a gene-environment interaction effect.

Despite these intriguing clues, the evidence for a unique epidemic of schizophrenia among certain immigrant groups, although suggestive, is not conclusive. No studies have controlled adequately for possible confounders such as low socioeconomic class and marital state, which may reduce the incidence ratio even further. It is likely that ethnicity represents a "proxy" variable for various social and perhaps biological factors. Once these are controlled, there may be little or no residual effect of ethnicity itself but we would gain information about other, perhaps preventable, risk factors involved. The most parsiminious conclusion would be that schizophrenia in immigrants is caused by the same factors that cause schizophrenia in other groups but that these factors are more common, (and therefore more conspicious), after migration. The alternatives—that there are specific causes in immigrants which do not occur in other populations or that there is true interaction with ubiquitious factors causing schizophrenia in only some groups—both require further research.

Course and outcome

Outcome studies in schizophrenia are usually based on hospital treatment samples and may not be representative of the population of schizophrenic patients[64]; indeed, the true natural course of schizophrenia is almost always masked by treatment these days. The results of outcome studies are difficult to summarise because the definitions of outcome and methods of assessment used are so varied. However, all studies attest to the striking variability of course and outcome of schizophrenia.[65] At the extremes of outcome, 20% of patients seem to recover completely after one episode of psychosis,[66-69] whereas 14%–19% of patients develop a chronic unremitting psychosis and never fully recover.[10 66 70] In general, clinical outcome at five years seems to follow the rule of thirds: with about 35% of patients in the poor outcome category[66 70]; 36% in the good outcome category,[66 71 72] and the remainder with intermediate outcome. Prognosis in schizophrenia does not seem to worsen after five years.[50 72]

The effect of changes in diagnostic criteria has been highlighted in a recent meta-analysis of outcome studies over 100 years,[71] which found that prognosis for schizophrenia has worsened over the past decade. The more restrictive definitions of schizophrenia post-DSM-III, predict worse prognosis, partly as a "self fulfilling prophecy", as chronicity over six months is already built into the definition of the disorder.[6]

Predictors of course and outcome

Immutable factors—Patients from developing countries have a better outcome than patients from developed countries,[10 66] but it is not known which aspects of non-Western culture are responsible for this effect. Possible social factors are lower levels of expressed emotion,[73] stronger social support networks, or lack of stigma. Ethnicity may be related to outcome but conclusions are preliminary.[74] Other favourable prognostic factors are good premorbid social adjustment, female sex, being married, and later age at onset,[10 66] but these factors are unlikely to act independently.[75] Acute onset of illness and the experience of negative life events before illness are also related to better outcome.[66 76]

Mutable factors—High levels of "expressed emotion" among close relatives—namely, criticism, hostility and overinvolvement[77 78]—predict early relapse. Substance misuse[10 79] also predicts poor prognosis. The important finding that delay in receiving treatment results in poorer outcome,[80-82] might be due to bias, and confounding with certain chemical characteristics resulting in delayed treatment, but it is possible that a more biological process is involved, with persistence of untreated positive symptoms altering the "hard wiring" in the brain.

43

Mortality

Standardised mortality ratios (SMRs) for schizophrenic patients are estimated to be two to four times higher than the general population,[83] and their life expectancy overall is 20% shorter than for the general population.[84] The most common cause of death (in 10% of patients), is suicide—the risk of suicide is 20 times higher than for the general population.[83 84] Young men with a chronic illness are at particular risk.[90] More work needs to be carried out to identify patients at risk of suicide, and to determine the effect of secular trends such as deinstitutionalisation on suicide rates. Deaths from heart disease and from diseases of the respiratory and digestive system are also increased among schizophrenic patients.[83 84] Certainly the lower socioeconomic status associated with schizophrenia carries with it many risk factors for physical diseases, such as smoking and poor diet, all of which are preventable.

Predisposition to violent behaviour

The association between schizophrenia and violence has received much public attention recently. A number of well-designed studies from the US and Sweden have found that the rate of violent offences is about 4–5 times higher among schizophrenic patients than among the general population.[84-88] These effects persisted despite controlling for factors such as social class, gender and educational level. Although it is important not to get the risk out of perspective it appears that there is a small but definite relationship between the diagnosis of schizophrenia and an increased risk for violence. It is likely that this applies to only a subgroup of patients and further research may help characterise those at higher risk for such behaviour.

Risk factors

Until recently, research into the aetiology of schizophrenia focused principally on family relationships and social stressors. A remarkable "paradigm shift" has taken place over the past decade; schizophrenia is now considered to be a brain disease and emphasis is placed on biological determinants.[91] The impetus for this change came from neuroimaging and neuropathological studies showing evidence of brain abnormalities in schizophrenic patients.[92] The timing of these pathological changes is unclear but is likely to be a defect in early brain development.[92] Profound changes have also occurred in hypotheses concerning neurotransmitter abnormalities in schizophrenia. The dopamine hypothesis has been extensively revised and is no longer considered a primary causative model—current research focuses on the interaction between different neurotransmitter systems.[93]

Genetic factors

Family studies

Schizophrenia runs in families. First degree relatives of schizophrenic patients have a morbid risk of developing schizophrenia which is 10 times higher than in the general population.[94 95] The excess risk of developing schizophrenia occurs principally among the children and siblings of patients. Parents are at lower risk of developing schizophrenia, probably because the low fertility associated with having schizophrenia means that parents are, of necessity, "selected for health", and have already survived much of the period of risk.[96] However, "familiality" of an illness does not necessarily indicate a genetic effect and can also be due to environmental factors. Adoption studies and twin studies allow these effects to be examined separately.

Adoption studies

Results from the influential Danish adoption study[97] show that the risk for schizophrenia among the biological first degree relatives of the schizophrenic adoptees is almost eight times higher than the risk among biological relatives of control adoptees.[98] Preliminary results from another large adoption study being carried out in Finland concur with these findings.[99] An increased risk of schizophrenia, in the absence of any contact with biological relatives, indicates that the familial aggregation of schizophrenia is due largely to genetic factors and not to some other aspect of the familial environment. Of course the adopted-away child has still spent the prenatal period with the biological mother and therefore prenatal environmental risk factors cannot be ruled out. However, the risk of schizophrenia spectrum disorders, (see below), was also increased in the paternal half siblings of the schizophrenic adoptees, who shared neither the prenatal nor familial environment.[97]

45

Twin studies

Twelve major twin studies of schizophrenia have been carried out, all of which show that the risk for schizophrenia in the co-twin of a schizophrenic proband (the *probandwise concordance*) is substantially higher for MZ than DZ twins.[100] Although the average probandwise concordance in MZ twins is 46% (compared with 14% in DZ twins),[101] the offspring of discordant MZ twins have *all* been found to share the same risk of developing the disorder,[102] raising the possibility that the unaffected MZ twin may represent an unexpressed genotype. Genetic factors are undoubtedly predominant but there is evidence (discussed below) that non-genetic factors may be involved in the aetiology of schizophrenia. The average estimate of the proportion of liability attributable to non-genetic factors in schizophrenia is 0·18.[100]

What is transmitted?

The "schizophrenia spectrum"—Certain psychiatric illnesses and personality disorders, known as the schizophrenia spectrum, are thought to be genetically linked to schizophrenia. The most important of these disorders is schizotypal personality disorder, and the relative risk for schizotypal personality disorder in the first degree relatives of schizophrenic probands compared with controls is about five.[103 104] Parents of schizophrenic patients have a higher risk of schizotypal personality disorder than siblings, suggesting that individuals who inherit this milder genetic vulnerability are responsible for the maintenance of schizophrenia in the population.[95] Within the cluster of symptoms and signs which comprise the diagnostic entity of schizotypal personality disorder—aloofness, poor rapport, social dysfunction, odd speech patterns, and avoidant symptoms in particular—predict genetic vulnerability to schizophrenia.[105]

Other disorders which form part of the schizophrenia spectrum are schizoaffective disorder,[106] paranoid personality disorder,[104] and schizoid personality disorder,[97 103] although there is some debate about the second.[104] No excess of anxiety disorder or alcoholism has been found in the relatives of schizophrenic patients compared with the relatives of controls, indicating that the genetic transmission of schizophrenia and schizophrenia spectrum disorders is relatively specific and does not include a generalised liability to all psychiatric illness.[97 103 107] The debate about whether affective disorders occur to excess in the relatives of schizophrenic patients has not yet been resolved,[94 107 108] although relatives of schizophrenic patients seem to have an increased predisposition to develop psychotic symptoms as part of an affective illness.[107]

Developmental abnormalities

Evidence for developmental abnormalities in schizophrenia has come from two sources of prospective data: (a) high risk studies and (b) general population birth cohorts.

High risk studies

The high risk study design involves following up offspring of schizophrenic mothers until they have passed through the period of risk for schizophrenia. Only the Copenhagen high risk study[109] has completed follow up of its probands, but because probands were recruited at age 15 there are no data on early development. The second generation of high risk studies in schizophrenia, which were started during the middle and late 1970s, began their observations on high risk children from the time of birth. The most influential of these studies are the New York High Risk Project,[110] the Jerusalem Infant Development Study,[111] and the high risk study of Barbara Fish.[112] As the subjects are now still in their teens and 20s, full information on outcome in the cohorts will not be available for another 10 years or so, but interesting data on infant and early childhood development among the high risk children have already been published and show a high degree of consistency between studies.

The developmental abnormalities found in 25%–56% of high risk children during different stages of childhood can be summarised as follows:

- *Neonatal period*: hypoactivity; extreme variation in alertness; hypotonia; poor "cuddliness"
- *Infancy*: a delay in acquisition of developmental milestones and a disordered pattern of acquisition of milestones— termed "pandysmaturation" by Fish[112 113]
- *Early childhood*: soft neurological signs, in particular poor motor coordination
- *Late childhood*: deficits in information processing and deficits in attention.

The question which remains to be answered is whether the children who have displayed these neurodevelopmental abnormalities throughout childhood will develop schizophrenia or a schizophrenia spectrum disorder in adulthood. Results from general population birth cohort studies (discussed below) and from a study based on examination of childhood "home movies" of schizophrenic patients[114] have replicated some of these developmental findings.

General population studies

Population based cohort studies can overcome the problem of generalisability associated with high risk studies. Unfortunately the information collected during childhood, although safe from selection and information bias, is often not ideal. In the United Kingdom, two such studies have now reported findings concerning schizophrenia.[40 41]

The National Survey of Health and Development, also referred to as the British 1946 birth cohort, comprises a sample of 5362 people born in the week 3–9 March 1946, who have been regularly followed up over four decades. Jones and colleagues[40] identified all cases of schizophrenia (30 in total) from this cohort and using the detailed, unbiased assessments made during childhood, investigated childhood developmental risk factors for adult schizophrenia in these patients using the remaining sample as a comparison group. Children who went on to develop schizophrenia as adults could be distinguished from their peers in the following ways:

- Motor development milestones, in particular walking, were delayed by an average of 1·2 months
- More speech problems (odds ratio/OR 2·8)
- Lower educational test scores at ages 8, 11, and 15
- Preference for solitary play at age 4 (OR 2·1)
- When the children were aged 4, health visitors rated the mother as having below average mothering skills and understanding of her child (OR 5·8): a finding which may indicate deviance in the child, the mother, or both.

The National Child Development Survey, also known as the British perinatal mortality survey, comprises all those born in the week 3–9 March 1958. Forty patients with schizophrenia were identified from this cohort. An investigation of childhood behavioural characteristics found that at the age of 7 patients were rated by their teachers as more socially maladjusted than controls.[41] Findings regarding low IQ were similar to the 1946 cohort.

These developmental findings are presumed to show differences in the way the brain is developing. Whether or not the developmental differences themselves modify risk, they have to be explained by any aetiological theory of schizophrenia, genetic or otherwise, and add a longitudinal aspect to the phenotype.

Non-genetic environmental risk factors

Birth complications

Case-control studies have found that schizophrenic patients as a group experience more birth complications than controls,[115] but studies may have been subject to many types of bias including recall, selection, and publication bias.[116] Three studies have used a cohort follow up design and have found modest increases in relative risk (about 2) for schizophrenia associated with certain birth complications: chronic fetal hypoxia,[117] low maternal weight,[118] and rhesus incompatibility.[119] However analyses from the 1996 Northern Finland birth cohort shows larger increases in risk for schizophrenia (between 4–6 fold) following CNS infections in early childhood,[120] and also suggest that perinatal hypoxia is a moderate risk factor. Furthermore, a recent case-control study based on standardised obstetric records from Scotland found an odds ratio of 9 for pre-eclampsia.[121] There is now good evidence that complications of birth and perinatal period contribute in some way to increasing the risk for later schizophrenia. Anoxic damage to the fetal brain may be the most important mechanism involved.

Place and time of birth

There is a small increase in risk for schizophrenia (OR 1·15), among people born in winter or early spring.[122] The reason for this season-of-birth effect is unknown, although it may be due to infectious diseases.[123] Being born in a city seems to be associated with a slight increase in risk for schizophrenia (OR 1·38), after adjusting for socioeconomic factors,[124] although not all studies have found such an effect.[40] Urbanisation, like social class, is a proxy measure for many other risk-increasing agents which are likely to operate synergistically.

Prenatal risk factors

Ecological studies have shown a modest increase in risk of schizophrenia (OR 2·0), associated with exposure to influenza in the second trimester of fetal life, particularly for the 1957 influenza epidemic.[125-127] Cohort follow up studies have had low power to examine this association,[128 129] and the case remains unproved. Nutritional deficiency during the first trimester may also increase risk (OR 2·0).[130 131] One intriguing, although unreplicated, study from Finland found that the risk of schizophrenia was higher (OR 6·2) among offspring of women who lost their spouse during pregnancy than for those whose spouse died during the child's first year, possibly indicating that severe maternal stress can affect fetal development.[132] Another recent Finnish study has found that individuals from the Northern Finland 1966 birth cohort who eventually developed schizophrenia were 2·4 times more likely to result from "unwanted" than "wanted" pregnancies even after adjustment for confounding by sociodemographic, pregnancy and perinatal variables.[133] "Unwantedness" may operate directly as a psychosocial stress during pregnancy thus increasing the risk for later schizophrenia. The true mechanism is quite obscure and a protective role for a propitious family environment is possible.

Heavy cannabis intake

Heavy cannabis consumption at the age of 18 was associated with an increased risk, adjusted for confounders, of later psychosis (OR 2·3) in a large cohort of military conscripts in Sweden.[134] A dose-response relation was convincing but the direction of causality remains in question.

Cerebral ventricular enlargement

Small case-control studies have been the mainstay of neuroimaging research in schizophrenia and findings are remarkably contradictory.[135] It is likely that the previously mentioned problems of bias, confounding, and inadequate power are at least partly responsible. The most consistent finding is that schizophrenic patients have larger lateral cerebral ventricles than controls. The level of risk associated with ventricular enlargement, adjusted for intracranial volume, age, sex, ethnicity, and social class, is about 2·0, although the whole notion of categorical definitions of pathology in terms of enlargement or shrinkage has been challenged.[136]

Risk factors as clues to aetiology

Examination of the effect sizes of various risk factors can give clues to causation. Table 2.1 shows that only genetic risk factors come anywhere near the effect size expected for a strong causal agent in schizophrenia. However, the existence of so many environmental risk factors with small effect sizes cannot be ignored. These may be proxy measures for an as yet unrecognised major environmental causal agent, or may act additively with each other or with chance events. They could also indicate the existence of gene-environment interactions.

Gene-environment interaction

Traditional aetiological models have considered vulnerability to schizophrenia as the sum of the impact of genetic and environmental risk factors—an additive model. But the concept of *gene-environment interaction*—that is, genes controlling sensitivity to the disease—predisposing effects of the environment, can no longer be neglected,[137] with many examples being found in the fields of medicine[138] and psychiatry.[139]

Both psychosocial and biological environmental factors may interact with genetic vulnerability to increase the risk for schizophrenia. Initial results from the Finnish adoption study of schizophrenia show a greater risk of psychosis among the

Table 2.1   Best estimate sizes of various genetic and environmental risk factors for schizophrenia (expressed as odds ratios or relative risks)

Category of risk factor	Specific risk factors	Best estimate of effect size
Genetic*	MZ twin of schizophrenic patients	46
	Child of two parents with schizophrenia	40
	DZ twin of schizophrenic patient	14
	Child of one schizophrenic patient	10
	Sibling of schizophrenic patient	10
	Parent of schizophrenic patient	5
Developmental†	Delayed milestones	3
	Speech problems	3
	Cerebral ventricular enlargement	2
Postnatal environment†	Immigrant/ethnic minority status	5
	Chronic cannabis consumption	2
	Solitariness as child	2
Prenatal and perinatal environment†	Birth complications	2
	Severe undernutrition (1st trimester)	2
	Maternal influenza (2nd trimester)	2
	Born in city	1·4
	Born in winter/early spring	1·1

*Relative risks; †odds ratios

biological offspring of schizophrenic mothers who were placed in poorly functioning adoptive homes than among those in well functioning adoptive homes.[99] High risk children who were reared in a kibbutz had increased rates of schizophrenia in adulthood compared with those who were reared in family homes, whereas control (low risk) children reared in a kibbutz had no increased risk of psychopathology.[140] A series of analyses from the Copenhagen high risk study has shown that birth complications may interact with genetic factors to increase the risk of schizophrenia.[98 141 142]

In other words, the pathogenic effects of birth complications, an adverse adoptive home, or some aspect of life in a kibbutz seem to increase risk of schizophrenia only in children who already have some degree of genetic vulnerability. Although the evidence is preliminary, it indicates that the environment should no longer be considered a "nuisance variable" by psychiatric geneticists. Common environmental factors may work in combination with rare high risk genotypes to maintain schizophrenia in the population.

New strategies in molecular genetics

The search for the "psychosis gene"[143] has met with substantial difficulties, including lack of a valid phenotype; the possibility of genetic heterogeneity; the possibility of environmental effects acting alone or in combination with genetic factors; and lack of knowledge about the exact mode of transmission.[100] Traditional linkage techniques are only able to exclude the existence of single major genes. As the genetic aetiology of schizophrenia is likely to be complex, involving genes of small effect, new techniques, and strategies are necessary.[96 100 143]

Linkage studies

Linkage strategies for detecting genes of small effect include non-parametric techniques, such as affected sib pair and affected relative pair approaches, which make no assumptions about mode of transmission. A recent variation on the sib pair design is the quantitative trait locus approach which involves measuring liability to schizophrenia as a continuous variable in siblings.[144 145] The application of the techniques of behavioural genetics to the study of schizophrenia is likely to prove a fruitful area for the future.[144]

After a false positive report of linkage on chromosome 5,[146] current interest centres on chromosome 22[147] and particularly on chromosome 6.[147] There is now strong, replicated evidence for the existence of a schizophrenia locus on the short arm (p) of chromosome 6.[148 149] The estimates of the fraction of each pedigree containing 6p-linked schizophrenics vary but 15–30% seems to be a close consensus. The region at 6p 21–24 contains maybe hundreds of genes and it will not be an easy task to narrow the search further. There is also moderately strong evidence for a susceptibility locus for schizophrenia on the long arm of chromosome 22.[150]

Association studies

Allellic association studies, which compare the frequency of marker alleles in a sample of patients compared with ethnically matched controls, are another method useful for examining genes of small effect.[146] An association between HLA A9 and schizophrenia has been found, but this effect is weak (OR 1·6), and its significance is uncertain.[96] Another promising area for the future is the use of newly developed DNA polymorphisms to examine candidate genes (genes coding for proteins which are likely a priori to be involved in the pathogenesis of schizophrenia)—for example, genes involved in neurodevelopment.[151] This approach offers the possibility of elucidating the cause of schizophrenia at a cellular level, bridging the gap between epidemiology and the basic sciences.

Conclusions

Schizophrenia occurs in all countries and in all races. On the whole, there is little variation in incidence or prevalence between countries, but there seems to be an increase in the incidence of schizophrenia when populations migrate. The reason for this immigration effect is unknown and is currently the subject of intensive study in the United Kingdom. Schizophrenia is associated with considerable morbidity and high mortality, and more information is needed on predictors of suicide among patients. However, on the positive side, the clinical outcome is not as hopeless as previously thought—almost 20% of patients make a full recovery after the first episode of psychosis and there is suggestive, although not conclusive, evidence for a decrease in incidence in the developing world.

The aggregation of schizophrenia in families, the evidence from twin and adoption studies, and the lack of variation in incidence world wide, indicate that schizophrenia is primarily a genetic condition, although environmental risk factors are also involved at some level as necessary, sufficient, or interactive causes. The persistence of schizophrenia in the population despite low fertility and high mortality, suggests that genetic transmission occurs principally through persons who do not have the illness. Further refinement of the diagnostic concept of the *schizophrenia spectrum* in both cross sectional and longitudinal terms will help elucidate the mode of transmission, and reliable instruments must be developed to detect these disorders in the community.

Areas of particular interest for the future are studies of risk factors and developmental abnormalities in those with known genetic vulnerability for schizophrenia—for example, siblings; the use of new molecular genetic strategies—including behavioural genetics—and the study of gene-environment interactions. If current progress in epidemiological and genetic research in schizophrenia continues, it is likely that the aetiology of this complex disorder will at least begin to be unravelled before the "decade of the brain" is over.

MC is supported by a Wellcome Trust Research Training Fellowship in clinical epidemiology.

1 Cooper JE, Kendell RE, Gurland BJ, *et al. Psychiatric diagnosis in New York and London.* Oxford: Oxford University Press, 1972.
2 American Psychiatric Association. *Diagnostic and statistical manual.* 3rd ed. Washington DC: APA, 1980.
3 American Psychiatric Association. *Diagnostic and statistical manual.* 3rd ed, revised. Washington DC: APA, 1987.
4 American Psychiatric Association. *Diagnostic and statistical manual.* 4th ed. Washington DC: APA, 1994.
5 World Health Organisation. *The ICD-10 classification of mental and behavioural disorders: diagnostic criteria for research.* Geneva, Switzerland: WHO, 1994.
6 Andreasen N. Changing concepts of schizophrenia and the ahistorical fallacy. *Am J Psychiatry* 1994;**151**:1405–7.
7 Plum F. Prospects for research on schizophrenia. 3. Neuropsychology. Neuropathological findings. *Neurosciences Research Program Bulletin* 1972;**10**:384–8.
8 Lewis G, Pelosi A. The case-control study in psychiatry. *Br J Psychiatry* 1990;**157**:197–207.
9 Wing JK, Cooper JE, Sartorius N. *The measurement and classification of psychiatric symptoms.* Cambridge: Cambridge University Press. 1974.

10 Jablensky A, Sartorius N, Ernberg G, *et al*. Schizophrenia: manifestations, incidence and course in different cultures. A World Health Organisation ten country study. *Psychol Med* 1992; monograph supplement 20.

11 Keith SJ, Regier DA, Rae DS. Schizophrenic disorders. In: Robins LN, Regier DA, eds. *Psychiatric disorders in America: the Epidemiologic Catchment Area Study*. New York: Free Press, 1991;33–52.

12 Kessler RC, McGonagle KA, Zhao S, *et al*. Lifetime and 12-month prevalence of DSM-III-R psychiatric disorders in the United States: results from the National Comorbidity Survey. *Arch Gen Psychiatry* 1994;**52**:8–19.

13 Office of Population Censuses and Surveys. *OPCS surveys of psychiatric morbidity in Great Britain*: bulletin No 1. *The prevalence of psychiatric morbidity among adults aged 16–64 living in private households in Great Britain*. London: OPCS.

14 Mason P, Wilkinson G. The prevalence of psychiatric morbidity. OPCS survey of psychiatric morbidity in Great Britain. *Br J Psychiatry* 1996;**168**:1–3.

15 Eagles JM, Whalley LJ. Decline in the diagnosis of schizophrenia among first admissions to the Scottish mental hospitals from 1969–78. *Br J Psychiatry* 1985;**146**:151–4.

16 Der G, Gupta S, Murray RM. Is schizophrenia disappearing? *Lancet* 1990;**335**:513–6.

17 Castle D, Wessely S, Der G, Murray RM. The incidence of operationally-defined schizophrenia in Camberwell 1965–84. *Br J Psychiatry* 1991;**159**:790–4.

18 Bamrah JS, Freeman HL, Goldberg DP. Epidemiology of schizophrenia in Salford 1974–1984. Changes in an urban community over ten years. *Br J Psychiatry* 1991;**159**:802–10.

19 Harrison G, Cooper JE, Gancarczyk R. Changes in the administrative incidence of schizophrenia. *Br J Psychiatry* 1991;**159**:811–16.

20 De Alarcon J, Seagroatt V, Goldacre M. Trends in schizophrenia. *Lancet* 1990;**335**:852–3.

21 Eagles JM, Hunter D, McCance C. Decline in the diagnosis of schizophrenia among first contacts with psychiatric services in North East Scotland, 1969–84. *Br J Psychiatry* 1988;**152**:793–8.

22 Kendell RE, Malcolm DE, Adams W. The problem of detecting changes in the incidence of schizophrenia. *Br J Psychiatry* 1993;**162**:212–8.

23 Geddes JR, Black RJ, Whalley LJ, *et al*. Persistence of the decline in the diagnosis of schizophrenia among first admissions to Scottish hospitals from 1969–1988. *Br J Psychiatry* 1993;**163**:620–6.

24 Munk-Jorgensen P. Decreasing first-admission rates of schizophrenia among males in Denmark from 1970 to 1984. *Acta Psychiatr Scand* 1986;**73**:645–50.

25 Munk-Jorgensen P, Mortensen PB. Incidence and other aspects of the epidemiology of schizophrenia in Denmark, 1971–87. *Br J Psychiatry* 1992;**161**:489–95.

26 Joyce PR. Changing trends in first admissions and readmissions for mania and schizophrenia in New Zealand. *Aus NZ J Psychiatry* 1987;**21**:82–6.

27 Nicole L, Lesage A, Lalonde P. Lower incidence and increased male:female ratio in schizophrenia. *Br J Psychiatry* 1992;**161**:557–6.

28 Waddington JL, Youssef HA. Evidence for gender-specific decline in the rate of schizophrenia in a rural population over a fifty-year period. *Br J Psychiatry* 1994;**164**:171–6.

29 Stoll AL, Tohen M, Baldessarini RJ, *et al*. Shifts in diagnostic frequencies of schizophrenia and major affective disorders at six North American psychiatric hospitals, 1972–88. *Am J Psychiatry* 1993;**150**:1668–73.

30 Oldehinkel AJ, Giel R. Time trends in the care-based incidence of schizophrenia. *Br J Psychiatry* 1995;**167**:777–8.

31 Jablensky A. Schizophrenia: recent epidemiologic issues. *Epidemiol Rev* 1995;**17**:10–20.

32 Keith SJ, Regier DA, Rae DS. Schizophrenic disorders. In: Robins L, Regier DA, eds. *Psychiatric Disorders in America*. New York: Free Press, 1991:33–52.

33 Asarnow RF, Asarnow JR. Childhood onset schizophrenia. *Schizophr Bull* 1994;**20**:591–7.

34 Castle D, Murray RM. The epidemiology of late-onset schizophrenia. *Schizophr Bull* 1993;**19**:691–700.

35 Van Os J, Howard R, Takei N, Murray R. Increasing age is a risk factor for psychosis in the elderly. *Soc Psychiatry Psychiatr Epidemiol* 1995;**30**:161–4.

36 Loranger AW. Sex differences in age at onset of schizophrenia. *Arch Gen Psychiatry* 1984;**41**:157–61.

37 Lewine RRJ. Sex differences in age of symptom onset and first hospitalisation in schizophrenia. *Am J Orthopsychiatry* 1980;**50**:316–22.

38 Häfner H, Maurer K, Loeffler W, Reicher-Rossler A. The influence of age and sex on the onset and early course of schizophrenia. *Br J Psychiatry* 1993;**162**:80–6.

39 Häfner H, Reicher-Rossler A, An der Heiden H, Maurer K, Fätkenheuer B, Löffler W. Generating and testing a causal explanation of the gender difference in age at first onset of schizophrenia. *Psychol Med* 1993;**23**:924–40.

40 Jones P, Rodgers B, Murray R, Marmot M. Childhood developmental risk factors for schizophrenia in the 1946 national birth cohort. *Lancet* 1994;**344**:1398–402.

41 Done DJ, Crow TJ, Johnstone EC, Sacker A. Childhood antecedents of schizophrenia and affective illness: social adjustment at ages 7 and 11. *BMJ* 1994;**309**:699–703.

42 Aro S, Aro H, Kesmäki I. Socioeconomic mobility among patients with schizophrenia or major affective disorder: a 17-year retrospective follow-up. *Br J Psychiatry* 1995;**166**:759–67.

43 Jones PB, Bebbington P, Foerster A, *et al*. Premorbid social under-achievement in schizophrenia: results from the Camberwell collaborative psychosis study. *Br J Psychiatry* 1993;**162**:65–71.

44 Tien AY, Eaton WW. Psychopathological precursors and sociodemographic risk factors for the schizophrenia spectrum. *Arch Gen Psychiatry* 1992;**49**:37–46.

45 Böök JA, Wetterberg L, Modrzewska K. Schizophrenia in a North Swedish geographical isolate 1900–1977: epidemiology, genetics and biochemistry. *Clinical Genetics* 1978;**14**:373–94.

46 Torrey EF. *Schizophrenia and civilisation*. New York: Jason Aronson, 1980.

47 Torrey EF. Prevalence studies in schizophrenia. *Br J Psychiatry* 1987;**150**:598–608.

48 Crocetti GJ, Lemkau PV, Kulcar Z, Kesic B. Selected aspects of the epidemiology of psychoses in Croatia, Yugoslavia. II. The cluster sample and the results of the pilot survey. *Am J Epidemiology* 1971;**94**:126–34.

49 Eaton WW. Update on the epidemiology of schizophrenia. *Epidemiol Revs* 1991;**13**:320–8.

50 Jablensky A. Schizophrenia: the epidemiological horizon. In: Hirsch S, Weinberger D, eds. *Schizophrenia*. Oxford: Blackwell Science, 1995:206–53.

51 Harrison G, Owens D, Holton A, Neilson D, Boot D. A prospective study of severe mental disorder in Afro-Caribbean patients. *Psychol Med* 1988;**18**:643–57.

52 Wessley S, Castle D, Der G, Murray R. Schizophrenia and Afro-Caribbeans. A case-control study. *Br J Psychiatry* 1991;**159**:795–801.

53 Thomas CS, Stone K, Osborn M, Thomas PF, Fisher M. Psychiatric morbidity and compulsory admission among UK-born Europeans, Afro-Caribbeans and Asians in central Manchester. *Br J Psychiatry* 1993;**163**:91–99.

54 King M, Coker E, Leavey G, Hoare A, Johnson-Sabine E. Incidence of psychotic illness in London: a comparison of ethnic groups. *BMJ* 1994;**309**:1115–9.

55 Van Os J, Castle DJ, Takei N, Der G, Murray RM. Psychotic illness in ethnic minorities: clarification from the 1991 census. *Psychol Med* 1996;**26**:203–8.

56 Selten JP, Sijben N. First admission rate for schizophrenia in immigrants to The Netherlands: the Dutch National Register. *Soc Psychiatry Psychiatr Epidemiol* 1994;**29**:71–2.

57 Odegaard O. Emigration and insanity. *Acta Psychiatr Scand* 1932; suppl 4.

58 Burke AW. First admission rates and planning in Jamaica. *Soc Psychiatry* 1974;**15**:17–19.

59 Hickling FW. Psychiatric hospital admission rates in Jamaica, 1971 and 1988. *Br J Psychiatry* 1991;**159**:817–21.

60 McGovern D, Cope RV. First psychiatric admission rate of first and second generation Afro-Caribbeans. *Soc Psychiatry* 1987;**22**:139–49.

61 Warner R. Time trends in schizophrenia: changes in obstetric risk factors with industrialization. *Schizophr Bull* 1995;**21**:483–500.

62 Eagles JM. The relationship between schizophrenia and immigration. Are there alternative hypotheses? *Br J Psychiatry* 1991;**159**:783–9.

63 Sugarman PA, Craufurd D. Schizophrenia in the Afro-Caribbean community. *Br J Psychiatry* 1994;**164**:474–80.

64 Hutchinson G, Takei N, Fahy TA, Bhugra D, *et al.* Morbid risk of schizophrenia in first-degree relatives of white and african-caribbean patients with psychosis. *Br J Psych* 1996;**16**:776–80.

65 Ram R, Bromet EJ, Eaton WW, Pato C, Schwartz JE. The natural course of schizophrenia: a review of first admission studies. *Schizophr Bull* 1992; **18**:185–207.

66 Leff J, Sartorius N, Jablensky A, Korten A, Ernberg G. The International Pilot Study of Schizophrenia: five-year follow-up findings. *Psychol Med* 1992;**22**:131–45.

67 The Scottish Schizophrenia Research Group. The Scottish first episode schizophrenia study. VIII. Five year follow-up: clinical and psychosocial findings. *Br J Psychiatry* 1992;**161**:496–500.

68 Tohen M, Stoll AL, Strakowski SM, *et al.* The McLean first-episode psychosis project: six-month recovery and recurrence outcome. *Schizophr Bull* 1992;**18**:273–82.

69 Geddes J, Mercer G, Frith CD *et al.* Prediction of outcome following a first episode of schizophrenia: a follow-up study of Northwick Park first episode study subjects. *Br J Psychiatry* 1994;**165**:664–8.

70 Shepherd M, Watt D, Falloon I, Smeeton N. The natural history of schizophrenia: a five-year follow-up study of outcome and prediction in a representative sample of schizophrenics. *Psychol Med* 1989; monograph supplement 15.

71 Hegarty JD, Baldessarini RJ, Tohen M, Waterman C, Oepen G. One hundred years of schizophrenia: a meta-analysis of the outcome literature. *Am J Psychiatry* 1994;**151**:1409–16.

72 Bleuler M. *The Schizophrenic disorders: long-term patient and family studies.* New Haven, CT: Yale University Press, 1978.

73 Leff J, Wig NN, Bedi H, *et al.* Relatives expressed emotion and the course of schizophrenia in Chandigargh: a two-year follow-up study of a first contact sample. *Br J Psychiatry* 1990;**156**:351–6.

74 McKenzie K, Van Os J, Fahy T, Jones P, Harvey I, Toone B, Murray R. Psychosis with good prognosis in Afro-Caribbean people now living in the United Kingdom. *BMJ* 1995;**311**:1325–8.

75 Eaton WW. Update on the epidemiology of schizophrenia. *Epidemiol Rev* 1991;**13**:320–8.

76 Van Os J, Fahy T, Bebbington P, *et al*. The influence of life events on the subsequent course and outcome of psychotic illness. A prospective study of the Camberwell Collaborative Psychosis Study. *Psychol Med* 1994; **24**:503–13.

77 Brown GW, Birley JLT, Wing JK. Influence of family life on the course of schizophrenic disorders. *Br J Psychiatry* 1972;**121**:241–58.

78 Leff J, Kuipers L, Berkowitz R, Vaughan C, Sturgeon D. Life events, relative's expressed emotion and maintenance neuroleptics in schizophrenic relapse. *Psychol Med* 1983;**13**:799–800.

79 Linzen DH, Dingemans PM, Lenior ME. Cannabis abuse and the course of recent-onset schizophrenic disorders. *Arch Gen Psychiatry* 1994;**51**:273–9.

80 Johnstone EC, Crow TJ, Johnson AL, MacMillan JF. The Northwick Park study of first episode schizophrenia. 1. Presentation of the illness and problems relating to admission. *Br J Psychiatry* 1986;**148**:115–20.

81 Wyatt RJ. Neuroleptics and the natural course of schizophrenia. *Schizophr Bull* 1991;**17**:325–51.

82 Loebel AD, Lieberman JA, Alvir JMJ, *et al*. Duration of psychosis and outcome in first-episode schizophrenia. *Am J Psychiatry* 1992;**149**:1183–8.

83 Mortensen PB, Juel K. Mortality and causes of death in first-admitted schizophrenic patients. *Br J Psychiatry* 1993;**163**:183–9.

84 Newman SC, Bland RC. Mortality in a cohort of patients with schizophrenia: a record linkage study. *Can J Psychiatry* 1991;**36**:239–45.

85 Swanson JW, Holzer CE, Ganju VK, Jono RT. (1990) Violence and psychiatric disorder in the community: evidence from the epidemiologic catchment area surveys. *Hospital and Community Psychiatry*; **41**:761–70.

86 Link BG, Andrews H, Cullen FT. The violent and illegal behaviour of mental patients reconsidered. *Am Sociol. Rev.* 1992;**57**:275–92.

87 Lindqvist P, Allebeck P. Schizophrenia and crime: a longitudinal follow-up of 644 schizophrenics in Stockholm; 1990;**157**:345–50

88 Hogkins S. Mental disorders, intellectual deficiency and crime. *Arch Gen Psychiatry* 1992;**49**:476–85.

89 Eronen M, Hakola P, Tiihonen J. Mental disorders and homicidal behaviour in Finland. *Arch Gen Psychiatry* 1996; 497–501.

90 Roy A. Suicide in chronic schizophrenia. *Br J Psychiatry* 1982;**141**:171–7.

91 Carpenter WT, Buchanan RW. Schizophrenia. *N Engl J Med* 994;**330**:681–90.

92 Weinberger DR. Schizophrenia: from neuropathology to neurodevelopment. *Lancet* 1995;**346**:552–7.

93 Davis KL, Kahn RS, Ko G, Davidson M. Dopamine in schizophrenia: a review and reconceptualisation. *Am J Psychiatry* 1991;**148**:1474–86.

94 Maier W, Lichtermann D, Minges J, *et al*. Continuity and discontinuity of affective disorders and schizophrenia: results of a controlled family study. *Arch Gen Psychiatry* 1993;**50**:871–83.

95 Kendler KS, McGuire M, Gruenberg AM, O'Hare A, Spellman M, Walsh D. The Roscommon Family Study. I: Methods, diagnosis of probands and risk of schizophrenia in relatives. *Arch Gen Psychiatry* 1993;**50**:527–40.

96 McGuffin P, Owen M, Farmer AE. Genetic basis of schizophrenia. *Lancet* 1995;**346**:678–82.

97 Kety SS, Wender PH, Jacobsen B, *et al*. Mental illness in the biological and adoptive relatives of schizophrenic adoptees. *Arch Gen Psychiatry* 1994;**51**:442–55.

98 Kendler KS, Gruenberg AM, Kinney DK. Independent diagnoses of adoptees and relatives as defined by DSM-III criteria, in the provincial and national samples of the Danish adoption study of schizophrenia. *Arch Gen Psychiatry* 1994;**51**:456–68.

99 Tienari P. Interaction between genetic vulnerability and family environment: the Finnish adoptive study of schizophrenia. *Acta Psychiatr Scand* 1991;**84**:460–5.

100 Kendler KS, Diehl SR. Schizophrenia: genetics. In: Kaplan HI, Sadock BJ, eds. *Comprehensive textbook of psychiatry VI.* Vol 1. Baltimore: Williams and Wilkins, 1995;942–57.

101 Gottesman II, Shields J. *Schizophrenia, the epigenetic puzzle.* Cambridge: Cambridge University Press, 1982.

102 Gottesman II, Bertelsen A. Confirming unexpressed genotypes for schizophrenia. Risks in the offspring of Fischer's Danish identical and fraternal twins. *Arch Gen Psychiatry* 1989;**46**:867–72.

103 Parnas J, Cannon TD, Jacobsen B, *et al.* Lifetime DSM-III-R diagnostic outcomes in the offspring of schizophrenic mothers: results from the Copenhagen high-risk study. *Arch Gen Psychiatry* 1993;**50**:707–14.

104 Kendler KS, McGuire M, Gruemberg AM, *et al.* The Roscommon family study. III. Schizophrenia-related personality disorders in relatives. *Arch Gen Psychiatry* 1993;**50**:781–8.

105 Kendler KS, McGuire M, Gruenberg AM, Walsh D. Schizotypal symptoms and signs in the Roscommon family study: their factor structure and familial relationship with psychotic and affective disorder. *Arch Gen Psychiatry* 1995;**52**:296–303.

106 Kendler KS, McGuire M, Gruenberg AM, *et al.* The Roscommon family study. II. The risk of nonschizophrenic, nonaffective psychosis in relatives. *Arch Gen Psychiatry* 1993;**50**:645–52.

107 Kendler KS, McGuire M, Gruenberg AM, *et al.* The Roscommon family study. IV. Affective illness, anxiety disorders and alcoholism in relatives. *Arch Gen Psychiatry* 1993;**50**:952–60.

108 Crow TJ. The continuum of psychosis and its genetic origins. The sixty-fifth Maudsley lecture. *Br J Psychiatry* 1990;**156**:788–97.

109 Cannon TD, Mednick SA. The schizophrenia high-risk project in Copenhagen: three decades of progress. *Acta Psychiatr Scand* 993;**370**:33–47.

110 Erlenmeyer-Kimling L, Cornblatt B. The New York high risk project: a follow-up report. *Schizophr Bull* 1987;**13**:451–62.

111 Marcus J, Hans SL, Auerbach JG, Auerbach AG. Children at risk for schizophrenia: the Jerusalem infant development study. *Arch Gen Psychiatry* 1993;**50**:797–809.

112 Fish B. Neurobiologic antecedents of schizophrenia in children. *Arch Gen Psychiatry* 1977;**34**:1297–313.

113 Fish B. Infants at risk for schizophrenia: sequelae of a genetic neurointegrative defect. *Arch Gen Psychiatry* 1992;**49**:221–35.

114 Walker E, Lewine RJ. Prediction of adult-onset schizophrenia from childhood home movies of the patients. *Am J Psychiatry* 1994;**147**:1052–6.

115 Lewis SW, Owen MJ, Murray RM. Obstetric complications and schizophrenia: methodology and mechanisms. In: Schultz SC, Tamminga CA, eds. *Schizophrenia: a scientific focus.* New York; Oxford University Press, 1989:56–9.

116 Geddes JR, Lawrie SM. Obstetric complications and schizophrenia: a meta-analysis. *Br J Psychiatry* 1995;**167**:786–93.

117 Buka S, Tsuang MT, Lipsitt LP. Pregnancy-delivery complications and psychiatric diagnosis: a prospective study. *Arch Gen Psychiatry* 1993;**50**:151–6.

118 Done DJ, Johnstone EC, Frith CD, *et al.* Complications of pregnancy and delivery in relation to psychosis in adult life: data from the British perinatal mortality survey sample. *BMJ* 1991;**302**:1576–80.

119 Hollister M, Laing P, Mednick SA. Rhesus incompatibility as a risk factor for schizophrenia in male adults. *Arch Gen Psychiatry* 1996;**53**:19–24.

120 Rantakallio P, Jones P, Moring J, von Wendt L. Association between CNS infections during childhood and adult onset schizophrenia and other psychoses. A 28-year follow-up. *Int J Epid* 1997 (in press).

121 Kendell RE, Juszczak E, Cole SK. Obstetric complications and schizophrenia: a case control study based on standardised obstetric records. *Br J Psych* 1996;**168**:556–61.

122 Bradbury TN, Miller GA. Season of birth in schizophrenia: a review of the evidence, methodology and etiology. *Psychol Bull* 1985;**98**:569–94.

123 Cotter D, Larkin C, Waddington JL, O'Callaghan E. Season of birth in schizophrenia: clue or cul-de-sac? In: Waddington JL, Buckley PB, eds. *The Neurodevelopmental Basis of Schizophrenia*. Georgetown: RG Landes Co, 1996:17–30.

124 Lewis G, David A, Andreasson S, Allebeck P. Schizophrenia and city life. *Lancet* 1992;**340**:137–40.

125 Mednick SA, Machon RA, Huttunen MO, Bonett D. Adult schizophrenia following prenatal exposure to an influenza epidemic. *Arch Gen Psychiatry* 1988;**45**:171–6.

126 O'Callaghan E, Sham P, Takei N, Glover G, Murray RM. Schizophrenia after prenatal exposure to the 1957 A2 influenza epidemic. *Lancet* 1991;**337**:1248–50.

127 Adams W, Kendell RE, Hare EH, Munk-Jorgensen P. Epidemiological evidence that maternal influenza contributes to the aetiology of schizophrenia: an analysis of Scottish, English and Danish data. *Br J Psychiatry* 1993;**163**:522–34.

128 Crow TJ, Done DJ. Prenatal exposure to influenza does not cause schizophrenia. *Br J Psychiatry* 1992;**161**:390–3.

129 Cannon M, Cotter D, Coffey VP, *et al.* Schizophrenia after prenatal exposure to the 1957 influenza epidemic: a follow-up study. *Br J Psychiatry* 1996;168:368–71.

130 Susser E, Lin P. Schizophrenia after prenatal exposure to the Dutch hunger winter of 1944–1945. *Arch Gen Psychiatry* 1992;**49**:983–8.

131 Susser E, Neugebauer R, Hoek HW, *et al.* Schizophrenia after prenatal famine: further evidence. *Arch Gen Psychiatry* 1996;**53**:25–31.

132 Huttunen MO, Niskanen P. Prenatal loss of father and psychiatric disorders. *Arch Gen Psychiatry* 1978;**35**:429–31.

133 Myhrman A, Rantakallio P, Isohanni M, Jones P, Partanen U. Unwantedness of a pregnancy and schizophrenia in the child. *Br J Psychiatry,* 1996; **169**:637–40.

134 Andreasson S, Allebeck P, Engström A, Rydberg U. Cannabis and schizophrenia. *Lancet* 1987;2:1483–6.

135 Chua SE, McKenna PJ. Schizophrenia—a brain disease? A critical review of structural and functional cerebral abnormality in the disorder. *Br J Psychiatry* 1995;**166**:563–82.

136 Jones PB, Harvey I, Lewis SW, *et al.* Cerebral ventricle dimensions as risk factors for schizophrenia and affective psychosis: an epidemiological approach to analysis. *Psychol Med* 1994;24:995–1011.

137 Kendler KS. Genetic epidemiology in psychiatry: taking both genes and environment seriously. *Arch Gen Psychiatry* 1995;**52**:895–9.

138 Khoury MJ, Beaty TH, Newill CA, Bryant S, Cohen BH. Genetic-environmental interactions in chronic airways obstruction. *Am J Epidemiol* 1986;**15**:65–72.

139 Kendler KS, Kessler RC, Walters EE, *et al.* Stressful life events, genetic liability and onset of an episode of major depression in women. *Am J Psychiatry* 1995;**152**:833–42.

140 Mirsky AF, Silberman EK, Latz A, Nagler S. Adult outcomes of high-risk children: differential effects of town and kibbutz rearing. *Schizophr Bull* 1985;**11**:150–6.

141 Cannon TD, Mednick SA, Parnas J, *et al.* Developmental brain abnormalities in the offspring of schizophrenic mothers. I: Contributions of genetic and environmental factors. *Arch Gen Psychiatry* 1993;**50**:551–64.

142 Cannon TD, Mednick SA, Parnas J, *et al.* Developmental brain abnormalities in the offspring of schizophrenic mothers. II: Structural brain characteristics of schizophrenia and schizotypal personality disorder. *Arch Gen Psychiatry* 1994;**51**:955–62.

143 Crow TJ. The search for the psychosis gene. *Br J Psychiatry* 1991;**158**:611–4.

144 Plomin R, Owen MJ, McGuffin P. The genetic basis of complex human behaviours. *Science* 1994;**264**:1733–9.

145 Chapman JP, Chapman LJ, Kwapil TR. Scales for the assessment of schizotypy. In: Raine A, Lencz T, Mednick SA, eds. *Schizotypal personality.* New York: Cambridge University Press, 1995: Ch 5.

146 Sherrington R, Brynjolfsson J, Petursson H, *et al.* Localisation of a susceptibility locus for schizophrenia on chromosome 5. *Nature* 1988;**336**:164–7.

147 Vallada HP, Gill M, Sham P, *et al.* Linkage studies on chromosome 22 in familial schizophrenia. *Am J Med Genet* 1995;**60**:139–46.

148 Peltonen L. All out for chromosome 6. *Nature* 1995;**378**:665–66.

149 Sham P. Genetic epidemiology. *Br Med Bull* 1996;**52**:408–33.

150 Gill M, Vallada H, Collier D, *et al.* A combined analysis of D22S278 marker alleles in affected sib-pairs: support for a susceptibility locus for schizophrenia at chromosome 22q112. Schizophrenia Collaborative Linkage Group (chromosome 22). *Am J Med Genet* 1996;**67**:40–5.

151 Jones P, Murray R. The genetics of schizophrenia is the genetics of neurodevelopment. *Br J Psychiatry* 1991;**158**:615–23.

3 Stroke

KAY-TEE KHAW

> - There are large differences in rates of stroke between countries.
> - Since the 1950s stroke mortality has been declining substantially in most countries. The countries of Eastern Europe are an exception.
> - Raised blood pressure is long established as increasing risk of stroke. A lowering of diastolic blood pressure by 5 mm Hg reduces risk by 30–50%.
> - Dietary factors, such as antioxidant vitamins and folate, are emerging as important determinants of risk of stroke. This has implications for prevention of cerebrovascular disease.

Stroke accounts for about 10% of all deaths in industrialised countries and is responsible for a vast burden of disability in the community. Once a stroke has occurred, treatment is largely focused on care and rehabilitation. However, there is evidence to suggest that stroke is potentially preventable. Firstly, there are large international variations in mortality from stroke and migrants between areas where the rates of stroke are different generally experience a change in risk; this implies that environmental factors may be more important than genetic susceptibility in determining risk. Secondly, many countries have experienced a steep decline in mortality from stroke in recent decades; although alterations in diagnostic fashion or certification practice might account for a small proportion of this decline, the most likely explanation seems to be changes in risk factor levels over time. Thirdly, epidemiological studies on causes of stroke have indicated that some of these are avoidable.

Stroke is often grouped together with coronary heart disease as cardiovascular diseases but there are substantial differences in the epidemiology of stroke and coronary heart disease. The most notable of these are the differences in time trends and the fact that the pronounced male excess found for coronary heart disease is not seen in stroke.

Definitions

The World Health Organisation defines stroke as "rapidly developing clinical signs of focal (or global) disturbance of cerebral function, with symptoms lasting 24 hours or longer or leading to death with no apparent cause other than of vascular origin".[1,2] Thus subarachnoid haemorrhages are included but not transient ischaemic attacks, subdural haematoma, and tumour or infection causing haemorrhage or infarction. Clinical diagnoses have been shown to be reliable.[3]

Most comparisons of stroke using routinely collected vital statistics rely on mortality rates. These have disadvantages including issues of diagnostic reliability, and variable case fatality which have been fully discussed elsewhere.[4,5] It is also not possible in mortality data to make accurate distinctions between the various stroke subtypes, in particular between haemorrhagic and thrombotic strokes. Morbidity and disability due to stroke are also of major concern, but few routine sources are likely to provide satisfactory data. A substantial proportion of people having a stroke die suddenly before reaching hospital or are cared for at home; hospital admission or discharge statistics depend on admission policies and accessibility and these vary enormously from country to country and over time. Most studies on incidence of stroke have methodological problems. When community stroke registers have been specially set up, as in the World Health Organisation (WHO) MONICA Project,[4] the evidence suggests that, for the purposes of international comparisons, there is good agreement between mortality rates in official statistics and stroke incidence registers. Time trends also need to be viewed with caution because of changing coding practices but again, many comparative studies have been conducted to examine the impact of these.

Case fatality

In the MONICA study, case fatality rates (defined as the proportion of events that are fatal within 28 days of onset) averaged about 30%, although they ranged from 15%–50%, with the lowest case fatalities in the Nordic countries and the highest in most of the Eastern European populations; there was no substantial sex difference in case fatality.[3]

Mortality by age and sex

Table 3.1 shows the mortality rates for stroke by age and sex in the United Kingdom. Rates rise sharply with increasing age. In marked contrast with coronary heart disease, in which there is a 5:1 male:female ratio at younger ages, there is no consistent sex differential in stroke mortality rates.

International comparisons

Figure 3.1 shows age-standardised stroke mortality rates in men and women for selected countries between 1991–2.[6] The highest documented rates are now seen in the countries of Eastern Europe and the former USSR. There is substantial international variation with men and women in the highest rate countries having about fivefold the rates in the lowest rate countries. Whereas men tend to have slightly higher rates than women, the sex differential does not compare with the pronounced male excess for coronary heart disease noted elsewhere. Figure 3.2 shows age specific rates for the United Kingdom, United States, and Russian Federation and indicates that the age standardised mortality comparisons reflect consistent differences over all age groups.

Time trends

Figure 3.3 shows time trends in stroke mortality from 1950 to 1989[6] and illustrates how these differ between selected countries. Japan, which had the highest rates in 1950–4, had an increase in mortality during the 1960s but then experienced a substantial decline; this trend was similar in men and women, although greater in men. Most other countries experienced a decline in mortality from stroke although others, particularly in Eastern

Table 3.1   Mortality rates/100 000 for stroke, United Kingdom 1992 (from WHO[6])

	Stroke mortality rate/100 000/age group				
	35–44	*45–54*	*55–64*	*65–74*	*≥ 75*
Men	7	19	79	291	1351
Women	7	17	55	230	1438

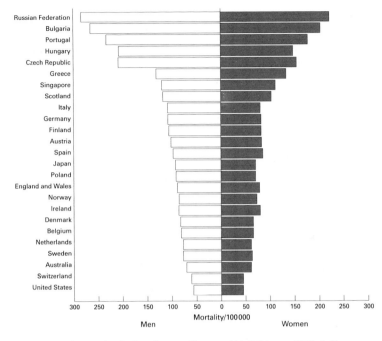

Figure 3.1   Age standardised stroke mortality rates 100 000 by sex 1990–2 (from WHO[6]).

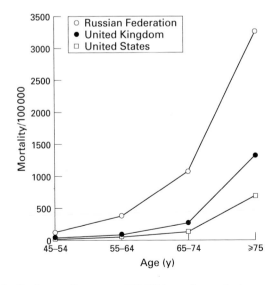

Figure 3.2   Stroke mortality rates per 100 000 by age for men in three countries.

65

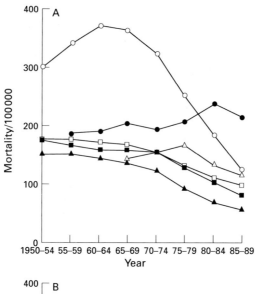

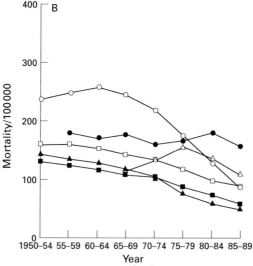

Figure 3.3 (A) Age standardised mortality rates 100 000 from stroke in men 1950–89. (B) Age standardised mortality rates 100 000 from stroke in women 1950–89.

○ Japan
● Hungary
□ England and Wales
■ France
△ Singapore
▲ United States

Europe—of which Hungary is an example—had an increase in rates and only from the 1980s was there a decline. The reason for these trends is unclear. It has often been noted that the decline in stroke mortality in the western countries preceded, and hence cannot be explained by, the use of antihypertensive medication.[7]

Figure 3.4 shows changes in stroke mortality rates between 1960–4 and 1985–9 in various countries. During this period many countries experienced substantial declines, more than halving stroke mortality; however, in some countries, notably those in eastern Europe, there was an increase in death rates. These trends suggest that the major determinants of mortality rates from stroke are likely to be potentially modifiable factors rather than genetic differences in stroke susceptibility. The results of migrant studies also emphasise this point; Japanese populations in the United

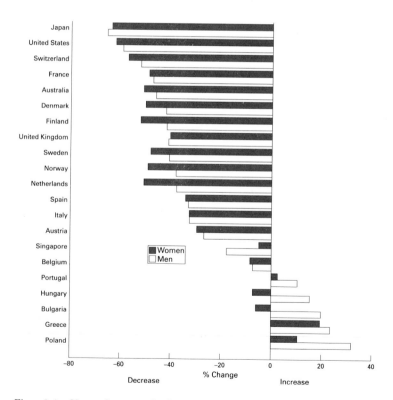

Figure 3.4   Changes in age standardised mortality rates from stroke in men and women 1960–4 and 1985–9 in selected countries.

67

States experience rates of stroke that are closer to those of American white populations than to those of Japanese populations in Japan.[8] Whereas some of the decline in stroke mortality may be due to a reduction in case fatality,[9] possibly due to better medical care or changing severity of disease, the magnitude of the declines suggest mortality rates also reflect changing incidence.

Regional and social class differences

Within any country, rates of mortality from stroke vary by social class and geographic region.[10] In Britain, rates vary over threefold between different regions, with the lowest mortality in the south and the highest in the north. Men in social class V have a risk of death from stroke nearly three times as high as men in social class 1; a similar pattern is seen in women.

Preventive strategies

There are two dimensions to the problem of stroke in the community: treatment, rehabilitation, and care of those who have had a stroke; and prevention of the occurrence of stroke. The large geographic variations, results of migrant studies, and changes over time in stroke mortality and incidence indicate the potential for prevention. Major challenges are to identify aetiological factors, and to quantify their potential impact on stroke burden. Laboratory, clinical, and epidemiological studies all contribute to our understanding of aetiology; this review focuses on the epidemiological evidence. Many biological and environmental factors have been implicated in the aetiology of stroke. Of these, the role of raised blood pressure has been the best documented. Strategies aimed at preventing stroke may be based on individual subjects or population based.[11] The high risk, or individual based approach aims to identify specific subjects at high risk of stroke for clinical interventions (such as that of reduction of high blood pressure using pharmacological therapy or behavioural changes). The population based approach aims to change levels of risk factors in the whole population to a more optimal distribution (such as by changing dietary patterns).

Biological risk factors

Blood pressure

The evidence for the aetiological role of raised blood pressure in stroke is overwhelming. Numerous prospective studies, recently reviewed,[12] have shown that systolic and diastolic blood pressure both independently predict stroke; the risk increases steeply and continuously with increasing blood pressure, with no threshold: the higher the blood pressure, the higher the stroke risk over the whole distribution of blood pressure, with relative risks increasing by nearly twofold for every 10 mm increase in diastolic blood pressure. Treatment trials of reduction of blood pressure have shown that a 5–6 mm Hg reduction in diastolic blood pressure reduces stroke risk by about 33–50%.[13]

Cholesterol

By contrast, the evidence that raised blood cholesterol, which is a powerful risk factor for coronary heart disease, has an effect on stroke is much more equivocal.[12] It has been postulated that the apparent lack of any consistent relation might be due to a positive association with ischaemic stroke and a negative association with haemorrhagic stroke; trials of cholesterol reduction to date have not had sufficient power to examine significant effects on stroke one way or another.

Other biological risk factors

Many other biological factors have been implicated as predictive of stroke. They provide intriguing evidence for the mechanisms underlying stroke and raise the possibility of preventive interventions. However, for these risk factors, there is as yet no evidence from intervention trials that changes in exposure will reduce risk of stroke. Raised fibrinogen,[14] raised homocysteine[15] and lower albumin concentrations,[16] raised white cell count,[17] infection,[18] poor respiratory function,[19] diabetes or impaired glucose tolerance,[20] and obesity, mainly central adiposity[21 22] have all been linked with increased risk of stroke. These factors may have independent effects, may interact, or may simply be markers of underlying processes. For example, white cell count or poor respiratory function may be a marker of chronic infection or inflammation, which may raise stroke risk by increasing the likelihood of thrombosis. Alternatively, white cell count might be a marker for cigarette smoking. Table 3.2 summarises these factors.

Table 3.2   Risk factors for stroke

Major risk factors	Prospective studies predictive of stroke	Intervention trial with stroke end point
Blood pressure	+	+
Cigarette smoking	+	−
Diabetes	+	−
Fibrinogen level	+	−
Obesity	+	−
Blood homocysteine level	+	−
Respiratory function	+	−
White cell count	+	−

Lifestyle risk factors

Many lifestyle factors have been linked with stroke (table 3.3). These include cigarette smoking, physical activity, and diet. Some prospective studies have reported direct associations between these factors and stroke mortality or incidence; the results of other studies suggest that dietary factors may influence risk of stroke by their effect on blood pressure.

Table 3.3   Lifestyle factors implicated in stroke

	Relation with blood pressure reported	Predictive of stroke in prospective studies
Diet:		
Adverse		
Sodium	+	−
Saturated fat	+	−
Alcohol	+	+
Protective		
Potassium	+	+
Vitamin C	+	+
Total calories	−	+
Fruit and vegetables	−	+
ω-3-fatty acids	+	−
Fibre	+	−
Cigarette smoking (adverse)	−	+
Physical activity (protective)	+	+
Obesity (adverse)	+	+

Smoking

Cigarette smoking is now well documented as increasing stroke risk; one study reported an approximate threefold risk in current compared with non-smokers.[23] It is not clear how smoking affects risk of stroke but it may be through thrombotic mechanisms.

Physical activity

Several studies have reported that physical activity is protective against stroke in both men and women[24-26]; this may be through influencing blood pressure, or through other mechanisms such as platelet aggregation.

Diet

Much interest and debate has focused on the role of dietary factors.[26-28] The evidence has been along two lines: dietary factors which may influence blood pressure, and thereby stroke, and dietary factors which may affect risk of stroke through other mechanisms, such as haemostasis or homocysteine concentrations. Of these, sodium has figured most prominently. The hypothesis that sodium might have an aetiological role in hypertension and stroke is not at all new but the debate is periodically revived.[29-33] There is little doubt from a wealth of intervention trials and observational studies that sodium has an effect on blood pressure; the debate is largely over the clinical and public health importance of the effect. Ecological studies have found that populations with a high sodium intake have an increased risk of stroke, but this association has not been convincingly demonstrated in prospective studies, perhaps due to the difficulty of measuring sodium intake. On balance, there is considerable circumstantial evidence that sodium is important in influencing hypertension and stroke risk. The magnitude of effect applied to the population has been estimated at about 10 mm Hg blood pressure difference for a 100 mmol difference in sodium intake, or about 34% difference in risk of stroke.[34]

Other dietary factors which have been related to blood pressure include potassium, magnesium, calcium, dietary fibre, ω-3 fatty acids, saturated fat, vitamin C, protein, and alcohol,[26 35-42] but again the relation with stroke is more uncertain. Several prospective studies have suggested that high intakes of potassium or vitamin C may be protective for stroke[43 44] and others that high alcohol intake may have an adverse effect, particularly as regards risk of haemorrhagic stroke.[45] Dietary factors may have effects other than on blood pressure. Antioxidant vitamins, for example, may influence haemostasis or endothelial function by protecting against free radical damage.[46] Folate may reduce stroke risk by influencing homocysteine concentrations. Fruit and vegetables are a rich source of vitamin C, potassium, and folate. Several studies have reported that a high fruit and vegetable intake seems to protect against stroke.[43 47–49] The magnitude of the effect was considerable with an estimated 25%–40% reduction in risk of stroke for an increase of two to three servings of fruit or vegetables daily.

Conclusions

Stroke is a devastating condition. However, the evidence from epidemiological and other studies suggests that stroke is eminently preventable; the challenge is to identify effective methods of prevention. We already have ample evidence that measures to reduce blood pressure in individual subjects and populations have a substantial impact on stroke rates. Because there is no threshold for the association with blood pressure, reduction of blood pressure in the population as a whole by altering lifestyle may be the most effective way to reduce the incidence of stroke. While the mechanisms remain to be clarified, intervention trials of vitamin supplements and other dietary modifications would be worthwhile. Such trials are already in progress in the USA. There is circumstantial evidence that lifestyle factors influence stroke risk in individual subjects and stroke rates in the community. Current health recommendations to increase fruit and vegetable intake, to reduce sodium intake, to increase physical activity, and to reduce cigarette smoking are likely to reduce risk of stroke and benefit health in general.

1 Tunstall Pedoe H, for the WHO MONICA Project Principal Investigators. The World Health Organisation MONICA Project (monitoring trends and determinants in cardiovascular disease): a major international collaboration. *J Clin Epidemiol* 1988;**41**:105–14.
2 World Health Organisation MONICA Project. *MONICA Manual, revised edition.* Geneva: Cardiovascular Diseases Unit, WHO; 1990.

3 Sandercock P, Molyneaux A, Warlow C. Value of computerised tomography in patients with stroke: the Oxfordshire Community Stroke Project. *BMJ* 1985;**290**:193–7.

4 Thorvaldsen P, Asplund K, Kuulasmaa K, Rajakangas AM, Schroll M. Stroke incidence, case fatality and mortality in the WHO MONICA Project. *Stroke* 1995;**26**:361–7.

5 Asplund K, Bonita R, Kuulasmaa K, *et al.* Multinational comparisons of stroke epidemiology. *Stroke* 1995;**26**:361–7.

6 World Health Organisation. *World Health statistics annuals 1982–1994*. Geneva: WHO, 1982–1994.

7 Klag MJ, Whelton PK, Seidler AJ. Decline in US stroke mortality. *Stroke* 1989;**20**:14–21.

8 Marmot MG, Syme SL, Kagan A, *et al.* Epidemiologic studies of coronary heart disease and stroke in Japanese men living in Japan, Hawaii and California: prevalence of coronary and hypertensive heart disease and associated risk factors. *Am J Epidemiol* 1975;**102**:514–25.

9 Bonita R, Beaglehole R. Explaining stroke mortality trends. *Lancet* 1993; **341**:1510–1.

10 Central Health Monitoring Unit. *Epidemiological overview series. Stroke. An epidemiological overview. The health of the Nation.* London: HMSO, 1994.

11 Rose G. *The strategy of preventive medicine.* Oxford: Oxford University Press, 1992.

12 Prospective Studies Collaboration. Cholesterol, diastolic blood pressure, and stroke: 13,000 strokes in 450,000 people in 45 prospective studies. *Lancet* 1995;**346**:1647–53.

13 Collins R, Peto R, MacMahon S, *et al.* Blood pressure, stroke and coronary heart disease. Part 2, short term reductions in blood pressure: overview of randomised drug trials in their epidemiologic context. *Lancet* 1990;**335**: 827–38.

14 Wilhelmsen L, Svardsudd K, Korsan-Bengten K, *et al.* Fibrinogen as a risk factor for stroke and myocardial infarction. *N Engl J Med* 1984;**311**:501–5.

15 Perry IJ, Refsum H, Morris RW, Ebrahim SB, Ueland PM, Shaper AG. Prospective study of serum total homocysteine concentration and risk of stroke in middle-aged British men. *Lancet* 1995;**346**:1395–98.

16 Gillum RF, Ingram DD, Makuc DM. Relation between serum albumin concentration and stroke incidence and death: the NHANES 1 epidemiologic follow up study. *Am J Epidemiol* 1994;**140**:876–88.

17 Gillum RF, Ingram DD, Makuc DM. White blood cell count and stroke incidence and death. *Am J Epidemiol* 1994;**139**:894–902.

18 Syrjanen J, Valtonen VV, Iivanainen M, Kaste M, Huttunen JK. Preceding infection as an important risk factor for ischaemic brain infarction in young and middle aged patients. *BMJ* 1988;**296**:1156–60.

19 Strachan DP. Ventilatory function as a predictor of fatal stroke. *BMJ* 1991;**302**:84–7.

20 Barrett-Connor E, Khaw KT. Diabetes—an independent risk factor for stroke? *Am J Epidemiol* 1988;**128**:116–23.

21 Shinton R, Shipley M, Rose G. Overweight and stroke in the Whitehall study. *J Epidemiol Community Health* 1991;**45**:138–42.

22 Welin L, Svardsudd K, Wilhelmsen L, Larsson B, Tibblin G. Analysis of risk factors for stroke in a cohort of men born in 1913. *N Engl J Med* 1987;**317**:521–6.

23 Khaw KT, Barrett-Connor E. Suarez L, Criqui M. Predictors of stroke-associated mortality in the elderly. *Stroke* 1984;**15**:244–8.

24 Gillum RF, Mussolino ME, Ingram DD. Physical activity and stroke incidence in women and men. *Am J Epidemiol* 1996;**143**:860–9.

25 Wannamethee G, Shaper AG. Physical activity and stroke in British middle aged men. *BMJ* 1992;**304**:597–601.

26 Manson JE, Stampfer MJ, Willett WC, *et al.* Physical activity and incidence of coronary heart disease and stroke in women. *Circulation* 1995;**91**:927.

27 Beilin LJ. Diet and hypertension: critical concepts and controversies. *J Hypertens* 1987;**5**:S447-S57.

28 Marmot MG, Poulter P. Primary prevention of stroke. *Lancet* 1992;**339**:344–7.

29 Bronner LL, Kanter DS, Manson JE. Primary prevention of stroke. *N Engl J Med* 1995;**333**:1392–400.

30 Frost CD, Law MR, Wald NJ. By how much does dietary salt reduction lower blood pressure: I: analysis of observational data within populations. *BMJ* 1991;**302**:815–9.

31 Elliott P, Stamler J, Nichols R, Dyer AR, Stamler R, Marmot M, *et al.* Intersalt revisited: further analyses from the Intersalt study on 24 hour urinary sodium and blood pressure. *BMJ* 1996;**312**:1249–53.

32 Thelle DS. Salt and blood pressure revisited. *BMJ* 1996;**312**:1240–1.

33 Khaw KT. Sodium, potassium, blood pressure and stroke. In: Poulter NP, Thom S, Sever PS, eds. Cardiovascular disease: risk factors and intervention. Oxford: Radcliffe Medical Press, 1993:145–52.

34 Law M. Commentary: evidence on salt is consistent. *BMJ* 1996;**312**:1284–5.

35 Swain JF, Rouse IL, Curley CB, Sacks FM. Comparison of the effects of oat bran and low-fibre wheat on serum lipoprotein levels and blood pressure.*N Engl J Med* 1990;**322**:147–52.

36 Criqui MH, Langer RD, Reed DM. Dietary alcohol, calcium, and potassium: independent and combined effects on blood pressure. *Circulation* 1989;**80**:609–14.

37 Harlan WR, Harlan LC. An epidemiological perspective on dietary electrolytes and hypertension. *J Hypertens* 1986;**4**:S334–9.

38 McCarron DA, Morris CD, Young E, Roullet C, Drueke T. Dietary calcium and blood pressure: modifying factors in specific populations. *Am J Clin Nutr* 1991;**54**:215S–9S.

39 Zhou B, Zhang X, Zhu A, *et al.* The relationship of dietary animal protein and electrolytes to blood pressure: a study on three Chinese populations. *Int J Epidemiol* 1994;**23**:716–22.

40 Salonen JT. Dietary fats, antioxidants and blood pressure. *Ann Med* 1991;**23**:295–8.

41 Obarzanek E, Velletri PA, Cutler JA. Dietary protein and blood pressure. *JAMA* 1996;**275**:1598–603.

42 Ness A, Khaw KT, Bingham S, Day NE. Vitamin C status and blood pressure. *J Hypertens* 1996;**14**:503–8.

43 Khaw KT, Barrett-Connor E. Dietary potassium and stroke-associated mortality: a twelve year prospective population study. *N Engl J Med* 1987;**216**:235–40.

44 Gale CR, Martyn CN, Winter PD, Cooper C. Vitamin C and risk of death from stroke and coronary heart disease in a cohort of elderly people. *BMJ* 1995;**310**:1563–6.

45 Gill JS, Zezulka AV, Shipley MJ, Gill SK, Beevers DG. Stroke and alcohol consumption. *New Engl J Med* 1986;**315**:1041–6.

46 Khaw KT, Woodhouse PR. Vitamin C, infection, haemostatic factors and cardiovascular disease risk. *BMJ* 1995;**310**:1559–63.

47 Gillman MW, Cupples A, Gagnon D, *et al.* Protective effect of fruits and vegetables on development of stroke in men. *JAMA* 1995;**273**:1113–7.

48 Vollset SE, Bjelke E. Does consumption of fruit and vegetables protect against stroke? *Lancet* 1983:**ii**:742.

49 Acheson RM, Williams DRR. Does consumption of fruit and vegetables protect against stroke? *Lancet* 1983;**i**:1191–3.

4 Head injury

BRYAN JENNETT

- Death rates from head injury in many countries are 2–3 times higher than those in Britain.
- Preventive legislation in developed countries has led to falls in death rates from head injury. In the developing world, rates are rising as road traffic increases.
- Risk of death or hospital admission for head injury peaks at 15–30 years. Rates in men are twice those in women.
- The causes of head injury vary with age. In children and the elderly, most head injuries are due to falls; at other ages, road traffic accidents, and in some places, assaults are the chief cause.

In western countries injuries are the leading cause of death under the age of 45 years, and in several Third World countries that applies also for ages 5–45 years. Because many injury victims are young, more years of life are lost in males below the age of 65 from trauma than from cardiac and cerebrovascular disease, or from cancer, in the United States, Japan, and several European countries.[1] Up to half of trauma deaths are due to head injuries but these account for most cases of permanent disability after injury.[2] Recognition that head injury is a major health problem has led to several studies over the past decade to produce epidemiological data in order to devise effective preventive measures, and to plan the most appropriate health care provision both for acute care and the rehabilitation of disabled survivors.

Limitations of available data

Reliable statistics are difficult to discover from routinely collected data. International comparisons of deaths from injury do not identify head injuries, although their incidence reflects geographical differences and trends over time in the frequency of trauma deaths as a whole. There are wide differences between countries in how many deaths are attributed to injuries, and how many injury deaths are due to motor vehicle or road deaths (table 4.1). The best time trend data are for road deaths and these have been falling for some years in many developed countries (table 4.2). This is believed to be mainly due to preventive measures such as seat belts, motorcycle helmets, enforcing laws on alcohol limits for drivers, speed limits, and improved car and road design. For example, in Great Britain the number of motorists tested for alcohol level in 1994 was 80% higher than the average for 1981–5, whereas the absolute number testing positive was halved; fatalities associated with drink driving were reduced by 70%.[5] Rates for road deaths are much higher in developing countries where such measures have not been taken (table 4.3), and are believed to be rising in such countries as vehicles become more

Table 4.1   Deaths from injury in different countries in 1985[3]

	Injuries as % of all deaths	Motor vehicle as % of injury deaths
France	7	30
Australia	5	51
United States	5	48
Canada	5	42
Japan	4	42
The Netherlands	3	41
Scotland	3	30
England	2	36

Table 4.2   Road deaths per 100 000 population[4]

	1980	1985	1993
France	21	20	17
Australia	24	18	—
USA	23	19	16
Canada	23	16	—
Japan	10	10	11
The Netherlands	13	11	8
Great Britain	11	9	7

Table 4.3   Road deaths per 1000 million vehicle km

	1985[6]	1993[4]
United States	15	9
United Kingdom	18	5
Japan	22	15
South Korea	540	—
Cameroons	530	—
Kenya (1984)	390	—
S Africa (1984)	180	—

common. In Taiwan deaths due to vehicle accidents rose from 31 per 100 000 population in 1977 to 37 per 100 000 in 1987[7]— higher than in any of the countries in table 4.2.

Data on hospital discharges and on deaths at national or local level do allow head injuries to be identified by the codes of the International Classification of Diseases (ICD) that specify location of injury. However, there are several difficulties in using these that limit the accuracy of data not only in routine statistics but also in research surveys that rely on ICD coding alone for case ascertainment. In the current (9th) edition of these codes[8] head injuries are covered by no less than 10 rubrics (table 4.4); moreover these are based on pathological rather than clinical criteria, and they are not mutually exclusive. For example, intracranial haematoma, the commonest treatable complication causing death and disability, is associated with skull fracture in 75% of cases, yet it is classified by a rubric that seems to exclude skull fracture. Severity of injury is also difficult to identify reliably from ICD codes. In particular the three digit codes make no reference to the duration or degree of impaired consciousness, the universally recognised clinical criterion of severity. More recently an expanded five digit clinical modification (ICD 9-CM) has been introduced which deals with the anomalies of fractures and haematomas and in a fifth digit registers duration of unconsciousness,[9] and this is now used in some United States hospitals. Another problem is the variation in the use of codes between hospitals when recording similar injuries, as well as simple coding errors. In one United States survey nearly two thirds of head injuries selected by ICD codes were excluded when the medical records were reviewed.[10] Therefore higher incidence

Table 4.4 *International Classification of Diseases*[8]

Three digit categories:

Fracture of skull, spine, and trunk (N800-N09)
N800   Fracture of vault of skull
N801   Fracture of base of skull
N802   Fracture of face bones
N803   Other and unqualified skull fractures
N804   Multiple fractures involving skull or face with other bones

Intracranial injury (excluding those with skull fracture):

N850   Concussion
N851   Cerebral laceration and contusion
N852   Subarachnoid, subdural, and extradural haemorrhage after injury (without mention of cerebral laceration or contusion)
N853   Other and unspecified intracranial haemorrhage after injury (without mention of cerebral laceration or contusion)
N854   Intracranial injury of other and unspecified nature

rates will be reported from surveys based on routine coding than when case records are reviewed. For example, Lyle et al[11] have suggested that the rate of 392 admissions per 100 000 population in New South Wales reported by Selecki et al[12] should be reduced to 266, to take account of the experience of Klauber et al in San Diego.[13] Incidence rates based on admissions (or discharges) may also be inflated by the double counting of patients transferred between acute hospitals (for example, from primary surgical wards to neurosurgical units and perhaps then back to primary surgical wards), and also by the inclusion of late admissions with delayed complications. Each of these has been estimated to account for 2% of recorded admissions for head injury.

Reports about head injuries from clinicians are of limited value. The several different specialists who are responsible for head injuries of different severities, together with varying admission and transfer policies in different places, make it difficult to put these reports into an epidemiological setting. The catchment population is often unknown, and the factors affecting the selection for treatment by a particular clinical unit are unlikely to be recognised, unless there are explicit policies. Most head injuries admitted to hospital are mild, but many clinical reports are from neurosurgeons who focus only on the 5%–10% of severe or complicated injuries that are transferred to them. Two large sets of data about severe injuries prospectively collected according to strict protocols from several centres are, however, now available. The international study of severe injuries that began in the Institute of Neurological Sciences in Glasgow in 1970 accumulated data from the Institute there and from centres in The Netherlands and California.[14 15] The United States National Coma Data Bank began 10 years later, collecting from four centres.[16 17] These two studies provide invaluable information about the minority of head injuries that are severe, but little about the population of head injuries from which they were selected or about the catchment populations. Reports from pathologists likewise focus on selected injuries, those from forensic laboratories including many victims who died instantaneously or very soon after injury. Such deaths that occur before admission to hospital account for two thirds or more of deaths from head injury in the United States and Australia and 45% of those in the United Kingdom. Reports from neuropathologists, by contrast, deal mostly with cases that survived long enough to be referred to specialist clinical centres, with very early deaths underrepresented.

Definition of head injury: grading severity

Head injury covers a wide range of severity from patients who die before admission to hospital to those with head injuries so mild that they do not even attend hospital. In between are those in coma, either initially or as a result of complications, those who are less serious but are admitted to hospital, and the much larger number who attend hospital but are sent home. Much of the difficulty in comparing different reports about the features and frequency of head injury stems from differing criteria for the minimum degree of severity required for classification as a head injury.

Most reports depend on administrative categories based on management or process, rather than on clinical criteria or outcome. The assumption is that cases admitted to hospital were more severe than those sent home, and that those transferred to a neurosurgical unit were more severe again. However, management policies, whether implicit or explicit, vary so much that the case mix of severity can vary widely from place to place. Policies can influence not only whether or not patients are admitted to hospital but also when they are discharged, so that duration of stay can be misleading as a measure of severity. Associated extracranial injuries can also distort the data by determining the admission, and prolonging the stay, of some patients. Social factors may have a similar influence—for example, for elderly patients and those who are injured far from home.

Clinical evidence of damage to the head is the most reliable way to recognise that a head injury has occurred, but all definitions exclude injuries confined to the face and foreign bodies in the nose or ears. Scalp, skull, or brain may each be injured independent of the other. Only 2% of attenders at Scottish accident departments for recent head injury have a skull fracture, but 15%–20% of severe and fatal injuries have no fracture.[18] Almost half of all attenders with head injuries in Scotland have a scalp laceration, but few have any evidence of brain damage by the time they arrive in hospital.[19 20] This applied to both adults and children and similar proportions have recently been found for a series of children in an American emergency room (personal communication). Some patients who are fully alert and oriented do, however, have a period of amnesia for some minutes after the injury. Most of the patients with head injuries admitted to hospital in Britain and the United States are only mildly injured. But a small minority of these patients develop complications—brain swelling or intracranial haematoma or infection. Moreover CT and MRI have recently confirmed what clinicians and psychologists have long suspected, that there is structural brain damage in some patients whose injuries seem to have been mild and who have not developed clinical complications.[21]

It has been suggested that patients who do not have either altered consciousness of a certain degree or duration, or neurological signs, should be excluded from estimates of incidence because they do not have *brain* injury.[22] In the light of the above clinical and imaging evidence the concept of "non-neurological" head injury seems to be unjustified on logical grounds, whereas it is certainly unwise from the standpoint of clinical management, as Fife[23] has also pointed out. These mild injuries are so frequent that they make considerable demands on the healthcare system, and they cause concern because of the small proportion who develop serious early complications, and the larger number who develop post-concussional symptoms. They are important also when exploring the pattern of causation of head injuries as a basis for devising strategies for prevention— because most mild injuries might well have been more severe, given only slightly different circumstances.

When milder injuries are included, as they are in most surveys, the incidence rates based on admissions are considerably higher than when only those with actual as distinct from potential brain damage are counted. Thus Kraus *et al*[22] recorded only 180 cases of traumatic brain injury per 100 000 population in San Diego in 1981 compared with an estimate of 295 in 1978 in a study that included milder cases.[13] Similarly, Lyle *et al*, applying the same exclusions to data from New South Wales, reduced the incidence from 266 to 180–200 per 100 000 population.[11]

Trauma centres now commonly use the abbreviated injury score (AIS) to define severity for trauma in general.[24] A conversion programme for deriving the AIS from the ICD 9-CM codes has been devised giving 5 severities: 1/2 minor, 3 moderate, 4 serious, 5 severe.[25] However, it proved much more difficult to convert the 519 possible combinations of head injury codes reliably to the five AIS categories than it did for injuries in other locations. The most common severity classification is by the Glasgow coma scale,[26] considering a score of 13–15 as mild, 9–12 as moderate, and 3–8 as severe. Others have used duration of unconsciousness or post-traumatic amnesia, but as post-traumatic amnesia is commonly as much as four times as long as the duration of coma these alternative definitions allow a wide latitude of severity. So also do the durations of altered consciousness used by different authors to distinguish mild from severe injuries. Durations of less than 15 or 30 minutes or 24 hours can count as mild, with severe defined as more than six or 24 hours of altered consciousness *or* evidence of brain contusion or intracranial haematoma. Classifications based on CT or MRI findings are suited only for the more severe injuries admitted to neurosurgeons.

Population based surveys in various countries

United Kingdom

Data for all deaths and for a 10% sample of admissions by ICD codes, and duration of inpatient stay have been published annually for many years in Britain, and these data for head injuries in England and Wales up to 1972 have been reviewed.[27] More detailed data for a stratified sample of injuries of all severities in Scotland in 1974 and 1985 have been analysed by an epidemiological team in Glasgow.[19 20 28–30] These studies included deaths before reaching hospital and attenders at emergency rooms sent home, as well as admissions to general hospitals and to neurosurgical units. The admissions included many patients without definite evidence of brain damage.

United States

Data on admissions for head injury are not routinely collected on a national basis in the United States, but discharges after head and spinal cord injury were reported from a sample of hospitals throughout the country during 1970–4.[31] Some local surveys have been reported since then and these have been reviewed by Jennett and Frankowski[32] and by Kraus.[2] A report of head injuries in Olmsted County, Minnesota from 1935–74 included deaths, admissions, and attenders but only those with loss of consciousness, amnesia, or neurological signs.[33] A survey in Bronx County in 1980 included admissions within 24 hours of an injury associated with unconsciousness of at least 10 minutes or skull fracture, neurological signs, or seizure.[34] Two surveys in San Diego identified cases by different criteria for 1978[13] and 1981.[22] The second was based on admissions with medically confirmed concussion or contusion and haemorrhage or laceration of the brain, and included prehospital deaths. A Chicago study compared two socioeconomically distinct communities: inner city and suburban; it included admissions within seven days of a blow to the head and all deaths were included.[35] A study of residents admitted to Rhode Island hospitals excluded early fatal injuries,[36] and the same went for a statewide study in Maryland.[37] Almost all these studies included cases of skull fracture without evidence of brain damage. A review of routinely collected mortality data from 1979–86 in the United States as a whole by the Centre for Disease Control identified deaths associated with head injury related to age, sex, race, cause, and region,[38] but acknowledged that these might have been underestimated by as much as 23%–44%—again indicating the limitation of routine statistics.

Other Countries

The epidemiology of neurotrauma (head, spine, and peripheral nerves) was studied in New South Wales, South Australia, and the Capital Territory of Australia in 1977 based on admissions and death records.[12 39] In Norway admissions after head injury to a regional hospital in 1979–80 have been reported[40] and also to a county hospital near Oslo for 1974–5.[41] A study in northern Sweden was limited to persons aged 16–60 years who had impaired brain function; it included early deaths.[42] In the region of Aquitaine in France all admissions and deaths after head injury were surveyed for the year 1986.[43] A study in Cantabria, Spain for 1988 was limited to admissions with loss of consciousness, skull fracture, or neurological signs, but excluded early deaths, which accounted for 92% of all deaths.[44] A study in Johannesburg was limited to admitted patients aged 15 years or over who had altered consciousness or evidence of contusion or laceration of the brain, excluding prehospital deaths.[45 46]

Variations in frequency of head injuries

Calculations of incidence vary according to whether the numerator is deaths, admissions, or attenders. They also depend on how well defined is the population denominator. Patients who were not local residents were excluded from some studies, but other reports suggested that they be included on the basis that they would be balanced by injuries sustained by local residents who were injured elsewhere during the same period.

Deaths

In several United States locations and in Australia, France, and Spain death rates from head injury are two to three times those in Britain (table 4.5). That for adults in Johannesburg is eight times greater than in Britain for all ages. The only reported rate that approached the low British level is that from a small sample of white patients in suburban Chicago.[35] In Britain the death rate from head injury has been falling since 1968[20] and was estimated to be only seven per 100 000 in 1994; a similar trend is reported from the United States.[38] Age specific mortality graphs are similar in Britain and one United States study (fig 4.1), but set at a higher level in the United States.[22] As in most countries for ages 15–60 years male rates are about twice those for females; the peak incidence is in males in the 15–30 age group.

The case fatality rates for those studies with population based rates for both admissions and deaths vary between 25.6% for Johannesburg to 3.2% for Scotland. They are higher when admissions are limited to cases with definite brain damage, when early death is excluded from incident rates based on admission, and when a large proportion of all deaths occur before hospital

Table 4.5   *Head injury admissions and deaths*

Place and reference	Year of study	Admissions/ 100 000	Deaths/ 100 000	Case fatality rate (%)
USA National[31]	1970–4	200	25	12.5
Olmsted[33]	1935–74	193	22	11.3
Bronx[34]	1981	249	28	10.8
San Diego[13]	1978	295	22	7.5
San Diego[22]	1981	180	30	16.6
Chicago[35]	1980			
City black		403	32	7.9
Suburban black		394	19	4.8
Suburban white		196	11	5.6
Australia[12]	1977	392	25	6.3
Australia[11]	1977	180–200	25	14–15.6
England[27]	1972	270	10	3.7
Scotland[20]	1974–6	313	10	3.2
Johannesburg[46]	1986	316	81	25.6
France[43]	1986	281	22	7.8
Spain[44]	1988	91	20	21.9
Northern Sweden[42]	1984	249	17	6.8

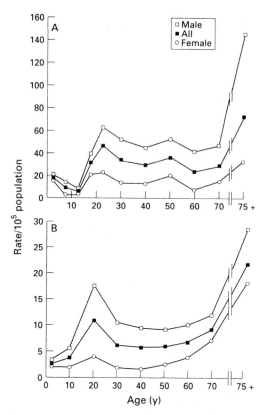

Figure 4.1   Age specific mortality rates for head injury. (A) San Diego 1981[22] (with permission); (B) England and Wales 1985.[47] Note the similarity in age distribution, with peaks in young adults and elderly people. The rates for San Diego are much higher at all ages than in England and Wales.

admission. Because many deaths occur before admission the in hospital case fatality rates are much lower (1%–6%) and are available for some studies that do not have population based mortality rates (table 4.6). The case fatality rates in clinical series of more severe injuries are much higher—14% for a regional neurosurgical unit in Virginia,[48] 15% for Scottish neurosurgical units,[30] and 33%[17] and 50%[15] for admissions in coma.

Admissions to hospital

Admission to hospital is a less reliable indicator of the incidence of head injuries because policies for admission vary widely even within one country, but they are an important indicator of the

84

Table 4.6   In hospital case fatality rates (CFRs)

Place and reference	Study year	Admission rate per 100 000	CFR (%)
San Diego[13 22]	1978	295	< 3
	1981	180	6
Maryland[37]	1986	132	4
Rhode Island[36]	1980	152	4.9
Norway[41 40]	1974–5	236	1.3
	1979–80	200	2.8
Sweden[42]	1984	249	1.3
France[43]	1986	281	2
Spain[44]	1988	91	1.7
Scotland[28]	1974	313	1.0

impact of local injuries on hospital resources. The age specific admission rates are very similar in Britain and the United States (fig 4.2) with a less dramatic rise in elderly people than in the mortality rates (fig 4.1). In Britain the regional range is 210–404 per 100 000 and for other countries 91–403 per 100 000 (table 4.5). However, most estimates are in the range of 200–300 per

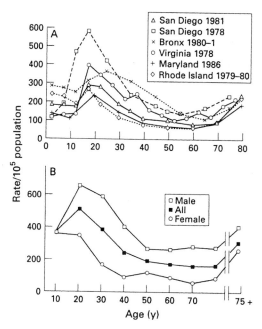

Figure 4.2   Age specific incidence rates (admissions) for head injury. (A) Various USA studies[2] (with permission); (B) Scotland.[49] The age distribution is similar in the two countries, and the rates are less different than for mortality.

85

100 000 despite differences in the criteria of severity used for case ascertainment, and the much wider variations in death rates. Moreover, despite these differences some 80% of admissions for head injury in most places are categorised as mild and only 5%–10% as severe. The mild cases are patients who were presumably admitted as a precaution against the development of serious complications. Thus two thirds of admissions to primary surgical wards in Scotland in 1974 had no skull fracture or evidence of brain damage and did not have an extracranial injury to account for admission. About 60%–70% of all admissions in United Kingdom hospitals were discharged within 48 hours. Publication of guidelines for admission triage in Britain[50 51] has led to some reduction in the proportion of attenders at accident and emergency departments that are admitted.[19] That fewer patients are admitted in the United States despite higher population mortality rates may be accounted for by there being access to neurosurgical advice in many more hospitals, giving other clinicians the confidence to send mildly injured patients home.

Patients with head injuries not admitted to hospital

Many patients with mild injuries either seek no medical attention or they attend hospital and are sent home after assessment. Data about such cases depend on specific surveys because no country keeps routine records of these cases. In 1974 about 20% of attenders with head injury in Scotland were admitted,[29] somewhat less than that a decade later.[19] This is very similar to a report of 20 years ago from Vancouver,[52] and recent findings for Rhode Island.[23] This last study estimated that during the years 1977–81 only 11%–22% (95% confidence interval) of head injured persons who were medically attended, or who reported at least one day of disability due to acute injury, were admitted to hospital. This indicated that cases not admitted to hospital accounted for 82% of all medically attended patients with head injuries in the United States, and for about half of all disability days due to head injury.

Some patients with minor head injuries may deliberately minimise or conceal their injuries. Sportsmen may worry that doctors will advise prolonged rest from their sport, and injuries associated with assault carry the risk of police investigation if a hospital becomes involved. Local geography and ease of access to medical care also influence whether or not mildly injured patients

Table 4.7   Attenders at accident/emergency departments
after head injury: age specific rates per 100 000 population
per year (Scotland 1985)[19]

	Children	Adults	All
All causes:			
All	4011	1473	1967
Males	5340	2180	2832
Females	2613	831	1158
Falls:			
All	2280	459	813
Males	2924	544	1035
Females	1603	381	605
Assaults:			
All	230	399	366
Males	350	677	610
Females	99	147	138
Road traffic accident:			
All	364	222	249
Males	486	306	343
Females	235	144	161

seek attention. These various factors combine to limit the accuracy of estimates of the incidence of head injuries as a whole. Indeed they can only be reliably counted when they impinge on the hospital system, or on the coroner or medical examiner. The number of patients who present at hospital after injury is, however, probably the best guide to the incidence, because this is least likely to be influenced by differences between health care systems, or local admission policies.

Incidence rates for attenders in Scotland in 1985 have been calculated on the basis of a countrywide survey (table 4.7). About half the attenders were children (under 15 years) giving an earlier peak incidence than for deaths or admissions (fig 4.3). Only about 20% of adults and 9% of children had any evidence of brain damage—either impairment of consciousness on arrival, or a history of brief post-traumatic amnesia or witnessed impairment of consciousness. In both adults and children 40% had a scalp laceration, which is more often found in those without brain damage. Incidence rates for those with brain damage were naturally much lower than for all attenders (table 4.8).

Disability and prevalence

A significant proportion of survivors of head injury are left with disability which may be both considerable and prolonged and it is of some importance to estimate the incidence and prevalence of such cases. Kraus[2] emphasises that even patients with mild injuries may be left with some disability for some months, and he

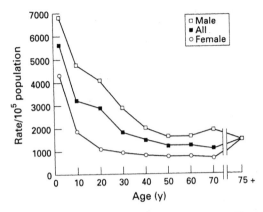

Figure 4.3 Age specific attendance rates for head injuries at Scottish accident and emergency departments for 1985[19] (with permission). About half the attenders are under 15 years, hence the earlier age for the peak of incidence rates than for deaths or admissions.

calculated that the number of new cases of disability from head injury per year in the United States varies from 33–45 per 100 000 according to whether 10% or 18% of patients with mild injuries are estimated as having some disability. Lyle *et al*[11] estimate on the basis of the San Diego study[22] that there are two per 100 000 new cases of severe disability and four per 100 000 of moderate disability per year there; he made a similar estimate for New South Wales. Because disability can persist for years the prevalence rates are much higher—one estimate for the United States was 439 per 100 000.[31] However, Moscato *et al*[53] in a household survey in Canada estimated 54 per 100 000 having at least six months of disability as a prevalence rate. The disability had lasted for more than five years in 65% of respondents and for more than 10 years in 45%. In a similar household survey in Scotland Bryden[54] found a prevalence rate of 100 per 100 000 for considerable disability, compared with an incidence rate of two per 100 000 of such newly disabled survivors.

Causes of head injury

All reports show that the main causes of head injury are road accidents, falls, and assaults. There is, however, considerable variation from place to place, with the proportion of admissions due to road accidents ranging from 24% in Scotland to 90% in

Table 4.8 Attenders with evidence of brain damage*: age specific rates per 100 000 per year (Scotland 1985)[19]

	Children	Adults	All
All causes:			
All	290	341	331
Males	395	537	508
Females	180	163	166
Falls:			
All	130	118	120
Males	165	168	167
Females	94	73	77
Assaults:			
All	6	147	78
Males	8	171	137
Females	4	26	22
Road traffic accident:			
All	99	70	76
Males	141	77	112
Females	55	39	42

*Brain damage = any evidence of altered consciousness either before or after reaching hospital, or neurologic signs.

Table 4.9 Distribution (%) of causes in different places (based on admission + early deaths)

Place and reference	Road traffic accidents	Falls	Assault
USA[31]	49	28	NI
Olmsted Co[33]	47	29	4
Bronx[34]	31	29	33
San Diego[22]	48	21	12
Rhode Island[36]	39	35	9
Chicago[35]			
City black	31	29	40
Suburban black	32	21	26
Suburban white	39	31	10
Maryland[37]	49	26	11
Australia[12]	53	28	NI
Scotland	24	39	20
France[43]	60	32	1
Spain[44]	60	24	NI
Taiwan[7]	90	5	NI
Johannesburg[46]	M 35	4	45
	F 39	3	38

NI = no information

Table 4.10 Main causes of head injury according to severity

	A and E attenders	PSW admissions	NSU transfers	NSU severe	Deaths
Year	1985	1985	1985	1984–6	1985
n	5242	1130	572	391	4100
Falls (%)	41	39	37	27	25
Assaults (%)	20	20	15	12	2
Road accidents (%)	13	24	32	50	58
Pedestrians as % of road traffic accidents (%)	29	39	46	50	-

A and E = Accident and emergency department (Scotland); PSW = Primary surgical ward (Scotland); NSU = neurosurgical unit (Glasgow); Severe = coma >6 hours (Glasgow). Deaths includes deaths at scene (England and Wales).

Taiwan (table 4.9). Similarly the proportion due to assault ranges from 1% of males in France to 45% of males in Johannesburg; in the United States the range is from 40% for inner city black persons in Chicago to 4% in Olmsted. The distribution of causes also varies greatly with the severity of injury, with road accidents the dominant cause only for severe and fatal injuries (table 4.10). Within a given severity there is also a pronounced·difference in the distribution of causes according to age and sex (tables 4.7, 4.8, and 4.11).

Among those with fatal head injuries from *road accidents* in the United States two thirds are vehicle occupants compared with only 40% in Britain, where pedestrians are often the victims. Pedestrians are apt to be more severely injured than occupants and injuries to pedestrians are particularly common in young children and elderly people. In Taiwan 62% of admissions with head injury from road accidents were motor cyclists, 33% were pedestrians, and only 5% were vehicle occupants. Clearly recommendations for preventive measures must take account of local conditions. There is increasing awareness of the importance of bicycle accidents, which are particularly common in children.[55-57] Most of the childhood accidents result from falls rather than collisions, and are often sustained off the road. It is often unclear whether they are included in road accident statistics or come under recreational activities.

Falls are a significant cause of head injury, particularly in young children and elderly people. Many falls in adults are related to alcohol and others result from assault, so that falls are likely to be underreported and the details are often inaccurate.

Assault is a common cause of head injury in some places, particularly in economically depressed and densely populated urban areas. In the Bronx[34] and inner Chicago[35] assault was the leading cause of head injury, but overall in the United States it accounted for only 10%. Within Rhode Island[36] and San Diego[58] rates of admission to hospital for head injury due to assault varied

Table 4.11 Causes of head injury admissions according to age and sex (Scotland 1985)

	< 15 y	15–64 y	> 65 y	Males	Females	All
n	351	653	117	785	336	1121
Falls (%)	55	27	40	35	49	39
Assaults (%)	5	32	3	34	12	20
Road accidents (%)	23	24	23	24	23	24
Pedestrians as % of road traffic accidents (%)	63	24	52	34	49	39

fivefold with deciles of median income. The frequency of gunshot wounds of the head in the United States is unique to that country, but there are wide regional variations there. There were 31 764 firearms related deaths in the United States in 1986, half of which were suicides and a third homicides; in some places gunshot wounds of the head account for half of all suicides and homicides.[59] Only 3%–6% of all admissions for head injury in the United States were due to firearms; they accounted for 20%–40% of all deaths from head injury in some local studies but for only 14% in the national deaths review.[38]

Alcohol is an important contributory cause of injury and its influence is best documented for road accidents, and especially for drivers. However, studies in New York city [60] and Glasgow[61] both showed that pedestrian victims of head injury were more often intoxicated than injured drivers. In San Diego over half the brain injured cyclists over the age of 15 were intoxicated.[55] Alcohol is also a common feature of victims of assaults, of falls, and of suicides. In admissions for head injury in Scotland alcohol featured four times more often after falls and assaults than after road accidents; in the latter pedestrians were affected twice as often as vehicle occupants.

Almost any *sport or recreational activity* can result in head injury. It is seldom clear from reports whether injuries ascribed to sport were limited to organised games, or also included informal recreational play. However, the importance of informal play as a cause of head injury in the young is highlighted in a recent report of 58 000 such injuries in United States emergency rooms.[62] Playground equipment and children's vehicles (excluding bicycles) were the main causes. In various United States studies some 10% of admissions for head injury were related to sport or recreational activities; in the Scottish survey 12% of new head injuries coming to emergency departments were attributed to sport.

Practical value of epidemiological data

Programmes directed towards reducing the number of head injuries, and minimising the damage to the brain when an accident does occur, have already had some impact. A strategy of prevention is, however, unlikely to realise its full potential unless there are reliable data about the incidence, demography, and geography of injuries in different places. Neither can the provision of medical services be planned appropriately without this knowledge. There is evidence that mortality can be reduced if there is a coherent scheme for the care of head injuries of all severities, but that most impact is made on less severe injuries.[63] Because mild injuries are so much more common, and among them are some patients who will develop serious but remediable complications, it is essential to have guidelines for the various specialties involved, to ensure that appropriate triage is carried out.[64] This is all the more essential in those countries where CT and neurosurgical services are provided on a regional basis. In those places secondary referral of serious injuries, and of mild injuries at risk of complications, is an essential component of good care for the community as a whole. Monitoring or audit of the care received and of the outcome depends on having reliable denominators. With increasing emphasis in all countries on the quality of care and on cost effectiveness it is important to ensure that reliable data are routinely collected about head injuries of all severities, their causes, and their outcomes.

1 Rockett IRH, Smith GS. Injury related to chronic disease: international review of premature mortality. *Am J Public Health* 1987:1345–7.

2 Kraus JF. Epidemiology of head injury. In: Cooper PR, ed. *Head injury*. 3rd ed. Baltimore: William Wilkins, 1993.

3 World Health Organisation. *1985 demographic year book: mortality statistics*. New York: United Nations, 1987.

4 Department of Transport. *Transport statistics Great Britain*. London: HMSO, 1995.

5 Report of Transport Road Accidents Great Britain 1994. *The casualty report*. London: HMSO, 1995.

6 International Road Federation. *World road statistics*. Geneva: IRF, 1988.

7 Lee S-T, Louis T-N, Chang C-N, Lang D-J, Heimberger RF, Fai H-D. Features of head injury in a developing country—Taiwan (1977–1987). *J Trauma* 1990;**30**: 194–9.

8 World Health Organisation: *Manual of the International Statistical Classification of Diseases, Injuries and Causes of Death*. 9th revision. Geneva: WHO, 1975.

9 Commission on Professional and Hospital Activities. *International Classification of Diseases*, 9th revision—*Clinical modification*. Ann Arbor, MI: Commission on Professional and Hospital Activities, 1980.

10 Anderson DW, Kalsbeek WD, Hartwell TD. The National Head and Spinal Cord Injury Survey: design and methodology. *J Neurosurg* 1980;**53**: S11–18.

11 Lyle DM, Quine S, Bauman A, Pierce JP. Counting heads: estimating traumatic brain injury in New South Wales. *Community Health Studies* 1990;**14**:118–25.

12 Selecki PR, Ring IT, Simpson PA, Vanderfield PK, Sewell MF. *Injuries to the head, spine and peripheral nerves Report on a study*. Sydney: New South Wales Government Printer, 1981.

13 Klauber MR, Barrett-Connor E, Marshall LF, Bowers SB. The epidemiology of head injury. A prospective study of an entire community—San Diego County, California 1978. *Am J Epidemiol* 1981; **113**:500–9.

14 Jennett B, Teasdale G, Galbraith S, Pickard J, Grant H, Braakman R, *et al.* Severe head injuries in three countries. *J Neurol Neurosurg Psychiatry* 1977;**40**:291–8.

15 Jennett B, Teasdale G, Braakman R, Minderhoud J, Heiden J, Kurze T. Prognosis of patients with severe head injury. *Neurosurgery* 1979;**4**:283–8.

16 Foulkes MA. Neurosurgical databases. *J Neurosurg* 1991;**75**:S1–7.

17 Foulkes MA, Eisenberg HM, Jane JA, Marmarou A, Marshall LF and the Trauma Coma Data Bank Research Group. The traumatic coma data bank: design methods and baseline characteristics. *J Neurosurg* 1991;**75**:S8–13.

18 Jennett B. Significance of skull X-rays in the management of recent head injury. *Clin Radiol* 1980;**31**:463–89.

19 Brookes M, MacMillan R, Culley S, Anderson E, Murray S, Mendelow AD, *et al.* Head injuries in accident/emergency departments. How different are children from adults? *J Epidemiol Community Health* 1990;**44**:147–51.

20 Jennett B, MacMillan R. Epidemiology of head injury. *BMJ* 1981;**282**:101–4.

21 Jenkins A, Teasdale GM, Hadley MDM, MacPherson P, Rowan JO. Brain lesions detected by magnetic resonance imaging in mild and severe head injuries. *Lancet* 1986;**ii**:445–6.

22 Kraus JF, Black MA, Hessol N, Ley P, Rokaw W, Sullivan C, *et al.* The incidence of acute brain injury and serious impairment in a defined population. *Am J Epidemiol* 1984;**119**:186–201.

23 Fife D. Head injury with and without hospital admission: comparisons of incidence and short term disability. *Am J Public Health* 1987;**77**:810–12.

24 Committee on Injury Scaling. *The abbreviated injury scale, 1985 revision.* Morton Grove, IL: American Association for Automedicine, 1985.

25 MacKenzie EJ, Steinwachs DM, Shankar B. Classifying trauma severity based on hospital discharge diagnoses: validation of an ICD-9CM to AIS-85 conversion table. *Med Care* 1989;**27**:412–22.

26 Teasdale G, Jennett B. Assessment of coma and impaired consciousness: a practical scale. *Lancet* 1974;**ii**:81–4.

27 Field JH. *Epidemiology of head injuries in England and Wales.* London: HMSO, 1976.

28 Scottish Head Injury Management Study. Head injuries in Scottish hospitals. *Lancet* 1977;**ii**:696–8.

29 Strang I, MacMillan R, Jennett B. Head injuries in accident and emergency departments at Scottish hospitals. *Injury* 1978;**10**:154–9.

30 Jennett B, Murray A, Colin J, McKean M, MacMillan R, Strang I. Head injuries in three Scottish neurosurgical units. *BMJ* 1979;**2**:955–8.

31 Kalsbeek WD, McLaurin RL, Harris BSH, Miller JD. The national head and spinal cord injury survey: major findings. *J Neurosurg* 1980;**53**:S19–31.

32 Jennett B, Frankowski RF. The epidemiology of head injury. In: Braakman R, ed. *Handbook of clinical neurology: 13 (57), Head Injury.* Amsterdam: Elsevier, 1990.

33 Annegers JF, Grabow JD, Kurland LT, Laws ER. The incidence, causes, and secular trends of head trauma in Olmsted County, Minnesota. *Neurology* 1980;**30**:912–19.

34 Cooper KD, Tabbador K, Hauser WA, Shulman K, Feiner C, Factor PR. The epidemiology of head injury in the Bronx. *Neuroepidemiology* 1983;**2**:70–88.

35 Whitman S, Coonley-Hoganson R, Desai BT. Comparative head trauma experience in two socioeconomically different Chicago-area communities: a population study. *Am J Epidemiol* 1984;**119**:570–80.

36 Fife D, Faich G, Hollinshead W, Boynton W. Incidence and outcome of hospital-treated head injury in Rhode Island. *Am J Public Health* 1986;**76**:773–8.

37 MacKenzie EJ, Edelstein SL, Flynn JP. Hospitalized head-injured patients in Maryland: incidence and severity of injuries. *Maryland Medical Journal* 1989;**38**:725–32.

38 Sosin DM, Sachs JJ, Smith SM. Head injury-associated deaths in the United States from 1979–1986. *JAMA* 1989;**262**:2251–5.

39 Simpson D, Antonio JD, North JB, Ring IT, Selecki BR, Sewell MF. Fatal injuries of the head and spine. Epidemiological studies in New South Wales and South Australia. *Med J Aust* 1981;**2**:660–4.

40 Edna T-H, Cappelen J. Hospital admitted head injury. A prospective study in Trondelag, Norway 1979–80. *Scand J Soc Med* 1985;**13**:23–7.

41 Nestvold K, Lundar T, Blikra G, Lonnun A. Head injuries during one year in a central hospital in Norway: a prospective study. *Neuroepidemiology* 1988; **7**:134–44.

42 Johanssen E, Ronnkvist M, Fugl-Meyer AR. Traumatic brain injury in northern Sweden. *Scand J Rehabil Med* 1991;**23**:179–85.

43 Tiret L, Hausherr E, Thicoipe M, Garros B, Maurette T, Castel J-P, *et al.* The epidemiology of head trauma in Aquitaine (France), 1986. A community-based study of hospital admissions and deaths. *Int J Epidemiol* 1990;**19**:133–40.

44 Vazquez-Barquero A, Vazquez-Barquero JL, Austin O, Pascual J, Gaite L, Herrera S. The epidemiology of head injury in Cantabria. *Eur J Epidemiol* 1992;**8**:832–7.

45 Brown DSO, Nell V. Epidemiology of traumatic brain injury in Johannesburg—1. Methodological issues in a developing country context. *Soc Sci Med* 1991;**33**:283–7.

46 Nell V, Brown DSO. Epidemiology of traumatic brain injury in Johannesburg—2. Morbidity, mortality and aetiology. *Soc Sci Med* 1991;**33**:289–96.

47 Office of Population Censuses and Surveys. *Mortality statistics: accidents and violence for England and Wales 1985.* London: HMSO, 1987 (Series DH4 (11)).

48 Jagger J, Levine JL, Jane JA, Rimmel RW. Epidemiologic features of head injury in a predominantly rural population. *J Trauma* 1984;**24**:40–4.

49 Scottish Home and Health Department. *Scottish hospital inpatient statistics 1985.* Edinburgh: Information and Statistics Division of the Common Services Agency, 1987.

50 Group of neurosurgeons: Guidelines for initial management after head injury in adults. *BMJ* 1984;**288**:983–9.

51 Teasdale GM, Murray G, Anderson E, Mendelow AD, MacMillan R, Jennett B, *et al.* Risks of acute traumatic intracranial haematoma in children and adults: implications for managing head injuries. *BMJ* 1990;**300**:363–7.

52 Klonoff H, Thompson GB. Epidemiology of head injuries in adults. *Can Med Assoc J* 1969;**100**:235–41.

53 Moscato BS, Trevisan M, Willer BS. The prevalence of a traumatic brain injury and co-occurring disabilities in a national household survey of adults. *J Neuropsychiatry Clin Neurosci* 1994;**6**:134–42.

54 Bryden J. How many head injured? The epidemiology of post head injury disability. In: Wood RLL, Eames P, eds. *Models of brain injury rehabilitation.* London: Chapman and Hall, 1989.

55 Kraus J, Fife D, Conroy C. Incidence, severity and outcomes of brain injuries involving bicycles. *Am J Public Health* 1987;**77**:76–7.

56 Thomson DC, Thomson RS, Rivira FP. Incidence of bicycle-related injuries in a defined population. *Am J Public Health* 1990;**80**:1388–90.

57 Sacks JJ, Holmgreen P, Smith SM, Sosin DM. Bicycle-associated head injuries and deaths in the United States from 1984 through 1988. *JAMA* 1991; **266**:3016–18.

58 Kraus JF, Fife D, Ramstein K, Conroy C, Cox P. The relationship of family income to the incidence, external causes, and outcomes of serious brain injury, San Diego County, California. *Am J Public Health* 1986;**76**:1345–7.

59 Fingerhut LA, Kleinman JC. *Firearm mortality among children and youth. Advance data from vital and health statistics.* No 178. Hyattsville, Maryland: National Center for Health Statistics 1989.

60 Haddon W Jr, Valien P, McCarroll JR, Umberger CJ. A controlled investigation of the characteristics of adult pedestrians fatally injured by motor vehicles in Manhattan. *J Chron Dis* 1961;**14**:655–61.

61 Galbraith S, Murray WR, Patel AR, Knill-Jones R. The relationship between alcohol and head injury and its effect on conscious level. *Br J Surg* 1976;**63**:138–40.

62 Baker SP, Fowler C, Li G, Warner M, Dannenberg AL. Head injuries incurred by children and young adults during informal recreation. *Am J Public Health* 1994;**84**:649–52.

63 Klauber MR, Marshall LF, Luerssen TG, Frankowski R, Tabaddor K, Eisenberg HM. Determinants of head injury mortality: importance of the low risk patient. *Neurosurgery* 1989;**24**:31–6.

64 Jennett B. Providing services for head-injured patients and auditing their effectiveness. In: Braakman R, ed. *Handbook of clinical neurology 13 (57), Head Injury.* Amsterdam, Elsevier, 1990.

5 Peripheral neuropathies

CHRISTOPHER MARTYN, RAC HUGHES

- There have been few population-based studies of peripheral neuropathies.
- Diabetes is the commonest single cause of peripheral neuropathy. Poor glycaemic control and duration of diabetes are the strongest risk factors.
- The annual incidence of Guillain-Barré syndrome is between 1–3 per 100 000. *Campylobacter jejuni* is the commonest recognized antecedent infection.
- The prevalence of hereditary neuropathies shows large geographical variations. The most frequent form is CMT1 which in about 70% of cases is associated with a duplication of the PMP22 gene on chromosome 17.

Peripheral neuropathy occurs as a component of several common and many rare diseases. It is heterogeneous in aetiology, diverse in pathology, and varied in severity. The term peripheral neuropathy includes symmetric polyneuropathy, single and multiple mono-neuropathy, and radiculopathy. Further classification depends on a mixture of phenomenological, pathological, and genetic or other aetiological features. All of these things cause problems for epidemiologists who, without agreed definitions of what constitutes a case, find it difficult to describe patterns of occurrence of disease. Perhaps it is not very surprising that information about the descriptive epidemiology of peripheral neuropathy derived from population based studies is scarce.

What data do exist suggest that peripheral neuropathy may be rather commoner than is usually thought. A recent study, carried out in two regions of Italy, estimated the frequency of chronic symmetric symptomatic polyneuropathy in people over the age of 55 years attending general practitioners' surgeries. Probable polyneuropathy was diagnosed if they answered positively to a screening questionnaire for neuropathic symptoms and showed signs compatible with peripheral neuropathy when examined by a

Table 5.1   Incidence of peripheral neuropathies

	Place	Incidence (per 100 000 person-years)	Reference
Bell's palsy	Minnesota, USA	25	83
	Texas, USA	23·5 men, 32·7 women	84
	Ehime, Japan	30	85
Cervical radiculopathy	Minnesota, USA	83	97
Guillain-Barré syndrome	Minnesota, USA	2·4 (1970–80)	27
	Farrara, Italy	2·7 (1991–3)	28
Carpal tunnel syndrome	Minnesota, USA	99	91
Neuralgic amyotrophy	Minnesota, USA	1·6	86

neurologist.[1] Around 8% of people met these diagnostic criteria for polyneuropathy. The commonest condition associated with polyneuropathy was diabetes. This study was not population based; only people already attending their general practitioner were included—a group in whom chronic disease is likely to be overrepresented and who will therefore be at increased risk of neuropathy. Despite this caveat, the rate of polyneuropathy detected was surprisingly high. Two studies of prevalence, one in Bombay[2] and the other in Sicily,[3] also suggest that peripheral neuropathy is common in the community. Cases were identified by a door to door survey. Those who answered positively to questions about sensory or motor symptoms were examined by a neurologist. In Bombay the prevalence of peripheral neuropathy was 2·4% and the commonest diagnoses were carpal tunnel syndrome and diabetic peripheral neuropathy. In Sicily, 7% of the population responded positively to the initial screening questions. After further investigation, diabetic neuropathy was diagnosed in

Table 5.2   Prevalence of peripheral neuropathies

		Prevalence (per 100 000 population)	Reference No
Overall	Italy	8000 (in people ≥ 55 y)	1
	Bombay, India	2400	2
Diabetic	Sicily	300	3
Carpal tunnel syndrome	Netherlands	5800 women, 600 men	90
Charcot-Marie-Tooth	Libya	8	15–21
	Nigeria	10	
	South Wales	17	
	Northern Sweden	20	
	Northern Spain	28	
	Western Norway	41	
Leprosy	South East Asia	116	65
	Africa	53	
	Central and South America	46	

0·3% but no details about the frequency of other types of neuropathy were published.

Peripheral neuropathies are a disparate group of diseases. Attempts to consider them as a whole emphasise their contribution to the burden of disease and disability in the community, but may obscure interesting epidemiological features that could lead to a better understanding of aetiology (tables 5.1 and 5.2). In this review we consider the commoner forms of peripheral neuropathy separately.

Diabetic neuropathies

The neuropathic complications of diabetes mellitus include distal, symmetric, predominantly sensory neuropathy, autonomic neuropathy, asymmetric proximal neuropathy, and cranial and other mononeuropathies. Several of these neuropathic manifestations may coexist in the same patient. Although the time course and prognosis of the different types of neuropathy vary, little is known about how this reflects differences in underlying pathology.

An early study of diabetic peripheral neuropathy in a population used retrospective review of case records to ascertain symptoms or signs of neuropathy.[4] Four per cent of diabetic patients developed peripheral neuropathy within five years of diagnosis. By 20 years after diagnosis, the prevalence had risen to 15%. Distal symmetric sensory neuropathy predominated. Many surveys since, both population based and of clinical case series, have shown that these rates are probably underestimates. Using a case definition that required at least two of the following three criteria—sensory symptoms in hands or feet, sensory or motor signs on examination, or absent or diminished tendon reflexes—a large registry based study of insulin dependent diabetic patients found an overall prevalence of distal symmetric polyneuropathy of 34%, which rose to 58% in people 30 years of age and older.[5] A study of non-insulin dependent diabetic patients, using criteria in which decreased or absent thermal sensation replaced sensory or motor signs, reported a prevalence of 26%.[6]

A recently published investigation in which a cohort of incident cases of non-insulin dependent diabetes mellitus was followed up for 10 years found that 8% fulfilled criteria for definite or probable neuropathy at the time of diagnosis compared with 2%

in the control group.[7] After 10 years of follow up, the prevalence of neuropathy had increased to 42% among diabetic patients and to 6% in controls. Electrophysiological investigations showed a more pronounced decrease in sensory and motor compound action potential amplitudes than in nerve conduction velocities in diabetic patients. This was interpreted as indicating that the underlying pathology was axonal degeneration rather than demyelination. Poor glycaemic control and low plasma concentrations of insulin independently of concentrations of glucose were associated with increased risk of development of neuropathy.

Lack of space prevents a detailed description of the many other studies that have been carried out but their findings are broadly similar. Poor glycaemic control and duration of diabetes have consistently been shown to be associated with neuropathy.[8] Other risk factors are age, height, male sex, and alcohol consumption although for these the evidence is less consistent. Systemic hypertension, cigarette smoking, and raised concentrations of plasma lipids are associated with increased risk of neuropathy in insulin dependent diabetes but not in non-insulin dependent diabetes. The central role of hyperglycaemia in the pathogenesis of diabetic peripheral neuropathy was confirmed in the large prospective Diabetes Control and Complications Trial. Intensive treatment of diabetes lowered the risk of developing clinical neuropathy by more than 60%.[9] Nerve conduction velocities were measured in over 1000 patients at entry to the trial and five years later. Significant differences were found between the intensive and conventional treatment groups. On average, the intensively treated group had faster sensory and motor conduction velocities and shorter F wave latencies than the conventionally treated group. Further, whereas most neurophysiological variables deteriorated over time among conventionally treated patients, they remained stable or showed modest improvement in the intensively treated group.[10]

Only one large population based study has investigated the prevalence of autonomic neuropathy in diabetes. Using three tests of autonomic function based on cardiovascular reflexes, the Oxford Community Diabetes Study found that nearly 17% of diabetic patients had at least one abnormal test.[11] Apart from erectile impotence, however, only 2·4% of the patients studied reported symptoms that could be attributed to autonomic dysfunction. Many other studies of clinic populations have also found that, whereas abnormal tests of autonomic function are common in diabetic patients, symptoms are relatively rare. There is some evidence to suggest that autonomic dysfunction in diabetes carries a poor prognosis. Mortality was high in two follow up studies of diabetic patients with abnormal tests of cardiovascular reflexes.[12 13] Autonomic neuropathy is a poor prognostic indicator in patients with advanced liver disease too.[14] This is an area that deserves further investigation.

Hereditary neuropathies

Charcot-Marie-Tooth disease is a heterogeneous group of disorders affecting the peripheral nerves and anterior horn cells of the spinal cord. Together they constitute the most commonly inherited form of peripheral neuropathy. Population surveys have been carried out which show large geographical variations in the frequency of the condition:[15-21] Libya 8 per 100 000 population; Nigeria 10 per 100 000; south Wales 17 per 100 000; northern Sweden 20 per 100 000; northern Spain 28 per 100 000; western Norway 41 per 100 000.

The most prevalent type is the demyelinating form, CMT1. In a study in northern Sweden, CMT1 accounted for 80% of cases whereas the axonal or neuronal form, CMT2, accounted for the remaining 20%.[19] A collaborative European study showed that about 70% of patients with CMT1 have an identifiable duplication of the gene for a 22 kDa peripheral nerve myelin protein PMP22 on the short arm of chromosome 17, at position 17p11·2.[22] In the others, various point mutations have been found in the PMP22, P0, and connexin 32 genes. The last is on the X chromosome and accounts for X linked cases. About 10% of families with autosomal dominant CMT1 have de novo duplications, usually, but not always, arising from duplication during male meiosis.[23] The severity of CMT is variable, even within families. Hereditary neuropathy may be subclinical, mild and late in onset, or severe from an early age. Hereditary neuropathy with liability to pressure palsies is an autosomal dominant condition, being due in most symptomatic cases (84% in the European collaborative study) to deletion of the same gene which is duplicated in the autosomal dominant subtype CMT1A at 17p11·2.[22] The phenotype is even more variable than in CMT1 and some cases are asymptomatic.

Amyloid neuropathy is the other common cause of hereditary neuropathy, being due to deposition of transthyretin, or less commonly other proteins, in the peripheral nerves, although it may also be an acquired disorder secondary to B cell dyscrasia and immunoglobulin light chain deposition. The nature of the mutation in the transthyretin gene determines the pattern of deposition and the presenting features of the neuropathy. The commonest mutation causes the substitution of methionine for valine at position 30 which results in a late onset, progressive, painful, predominantly sensory neuropathy, formerly called the Portuguese type or familial amyloid neuropathy type 1. It has been described from many different countries, including Portugal, Japan, Italy, Spain, Greece, and Sweden. There are few data on prevalence but published studies suggest that clusters of high prevalence occur in some areas. In northern Sweden the gene prevalence is 1500 per 100 000 but the disease is so mild and late in onset—or the penetrance so low—that the prevalence of symptomatic disease is only 31 per 100 000.[24] Studies of transthyretin intron polymorphisms have shown that there are multiple haplotypes, refuting the proposition that the disease had a single founder and was then spread round the world by Portuguese sailors.[25]

Neuropathy from infectious and inflammatory causes

Guillain-Barré syndrome

Guillain-Barré syndrome (GBS) has been the subject of over 30 population studies during the past 50 years, most of which have shown an annual incidence in the range 1·0 to 2·0 per 100 000 population. The condition seems to be reasonably evenly distributed throughout the world and incidence rates are probably fairly stable over time.[26] The annual incidence seemed to rise from 1·2 per 100 000 in 1953–6 to 2·7 per 100 000 in 1970–80 in Olmsted county, Rochester, USA.[27] Similarly the annual incidence rose from about 1·3 per 100 000 in the triennium 1981–3 to 2·7 per 100 000 in 1991–3 when surveyed in Ferrara, northern Italy.[28] These apparent increases in incidence were based on few cases and may be explained by increasing awareness and ascertainment of the disease.[28]

101

Whereas the incidence of GBS is low (but not very low, being about half that of multiple sclerosis), the cumulative effect of permanent disability produced in young people represents an important, but unrecognised public health problem. Thirteen per cent of 79 patients in a recent population based survey in south east England were left requiring aid to walk after a year, a disability likely to be permanent.[29]

The heterogeneity of GBS and lack of a gold standard diagnostic test bedevil useful aetiological deductions from population based surveys of the disease. In practice, the clinical picture is sufficiently striking that the diagnosis can be readily recognised in a community with ready access to neurological services and most cases conform to the accepted diagnostic criteria.[30] Unfortunately this clinical description embraces a heterogeneous group of pathological entities, of which at least 90% are thought to be acute inflammatory demyelinating polyradiculoneuropathy and the remainder are acute motor, or motor and sensory, axonal neuropathy.[31] None of the population based studies has been sufficiently complex to distinguish the different subtypes of GBS.

The disease occurs from infancy to extreme old age. There is a more or less linear increase in incidence with advancing years which would be compatible with lessening of immune suppressor mechanisms in old age and consequent increased susceptibility to autoimmune disease. In the largest series, collected in an active surveillance programme in the United States from 1979 to 1981, there was a small peak in the age distribution for young adults, especially women.[32] This might be explained by exposure to infections which are more common in that age group, which include *Campylobacter jejuni* and cytomegalovirus.

Males are more commonly affected than females in a ratio of 1·25 to 1.[33] Such male predominance is unusual for an autoimmune disease, but also occurs in Goodpasture's syndrome, which is due to autoantibodies against glomerular basement membrane. It is not clear whether this male predominant sex ratio is confined to the premenopausal age and explicable by a protective effect of oestrogen or to an X or Y chromosome gene. Such effects might operate at the level of susceptibility to an infection or control of an autoimmune response. The effect of sex on both factors has been shown in relevant experimental models. For instance, female mice experimentally infected with vesicular stomatitis virus developed less CNS virus load and recovered more quickly than males: the recovery was associated with an earlier, more vigorous inflammatory response.[34]

The occurrence of GBS is sporadic although rare, small epidemics have been reported.[35] For instance, an outbreak of nearly 4000 cases of gastroenteritis in a town in Jordan, attributed to *Shigella* contamination of the water, resulted in 19 cases of GBS, representing about four cases per 1000 reported cases of shigellosis.[36] There is no consistent seasonal pattern of incidence except in north China where there is a large increase in incidence of GBS in the summer months. This summer epidemic is due to an increase in incidence of acute motor axonal neuropathy in children and young adults.[37] Such a pattern strongly suggests exposure to a seasonal infection in the pathogenesis of this type of GBS in that region. The most likely candidate is *Campylobacter jejuni* enteritis: 66% of 38 cases had serological evidence of recent infection compared with 16% of village controls.[38] *Campylobacter jejuni* is also the commonest identified infection preceding sporadic GBS in other countries. In large series of cases of GBS (n > 100) in the United Kingdom,[31 39] The Netherlands,[40] and the United States,[41] the frequency of serological evidence of recent *Campylobacter* infection has ranged from 26 to 36% of cases of GBS, far exceeding the incidence in control groups,[31 39] and making *Campylobacter* the commonest recognised antecedent infection. The favoured hypothesis is that *Campylobacter* lipopolysaccharide glycoconjugates share epitopes with axonal or Schwann cell glycolipids, stimulate autoimmune responses, and generate corresponding axonal or demyelinating autoimmune neuropathy. In particular the Gal(β1–3) GalNAc epitope is shared by the lipopolysaccharide in the walls of some *Campylobacter* strains and by ganglioside GM1 in axon membranes.[42 43] Although the general hypothesis that *Campylobacter* infections stimulate immune responses to cross reactive glyconjugates may still be correct, ganglioside GM1-like epitopes are not invariably present in the lipopolysaccharide prepared from *Campylobacter* isolated from the stools of patients with GBS.[44] There is a single report, needing confirmation, of induction of acute axonal neuropathy in chickens which had been fed or injected with *Campylobacter* isolated from the stool of a Chinese patient with the acute motor axonal neuropathy form of GBS.[45]

There have been many single reports, and also small series of cases of GBS after therapeutic injection of ganglioside preparations.[46–48] Many, but not all, of the affected patients have had antibodies to ganglioside GM1 in their serum. There was no rise in the incidence of GBS after the introduction of ganglioside treatment during ongoing epidemiological surveys of GBS in Italy. Case-control studies have not proved a causal connection but the circumstantial evidence is strong.[49]

GBS is such a striking illness that when it occurs after an event such as an immunisation, it tends to be reported either in the medical literature or in the law courts. With the exception of vaccinia, the old fashioned rabies vaccines, which contained myelin components,[50] and the 1976 United States swine influenza vaccine,[51] the evidence that immunisations trigger GBS is not strong. However, disproving small increases in risk is difficult in diseases as uncommon as GBS. In two case control studies, comprising over 200 cases in south east England, the odds ratio of cases having been immunised was 1·8, not significantly increased compared with controls, but the 95% confidence intervals ranged from 0·7 to 4·4.[52] The epidemiologically demonstrated association between swine influenza vaccine and GBS was never explained. Ongoing investigations of the association with *Campylobacter* have already contributed to the description of the acute axonal motor and motor and sensory subtypes of GBS and may well yield the secret of how a bacterial infection can give rise to an autoimmune reaction directed against axonal or Schwann cell derived antigens.

Large series, population studies, and large controlled trials have consistently shown the following to be adverse prognostic factors: old age, preceding gastrointestinal infection, serological or stool culture evidence of *Campylobacter* infection, severe acute illness (requirement for ventilation or severe upper limb weakness), electrophysiological evidence of axonal degeneration (small distally evoked muscle action potentials), and absence of treatment with plasma exchange or intravenous immunoglobulin.[31 40 53 54]

Chronic inflammatory demyelinating polyradiculoneuropathy (CIDP)

By contrast with GBS there is very little epidemiological information concerning CIDP (defined as an acquired idiopathic demyelinating neuropathy with a progressive phase > eight weeks). The distinction between the acute inflammatory demyelinating polyradiculoneuropathy form of GBS and CIDP may be artificial as the distribution of onset phases is unimodal, not bimodal,[55] and intermediate subacute forms occur.[56] It is probably an uncommon condition but the neurophysiological and nerve biopsy assessments required for its diagnosis are complex so that it is probably underdiagnosed. There are no reliable population estimates of its prevalence yet, but our own data suggest a minimum prevalence of at least 1 per 100 000. The only published information at present comes from large hospital series which suggest that the disease occurs throughout the world and at all ages. Its course is more often relapsing-remitting than progressive, and progressive cases tend to be older.[57] Antecedent infections are reported less commonly than before GBS, being recalled in only 25% of 40 patients in the most recent study in which this information was specifically sought.[58] Although immunisations have also been incriminated as triggering CIDP, the evidence that they either trigger CIDP or cause relapse is weak.[59]

HIV associated neuropathy

Various peripheral nerve syndromes have been reported in association with HIV infection including acute and chronic inflammatory demyelinating neuropathies, distal sensory neuropathy—often of a painful type—and multiple mono-neuropathy. In addition, treatment with dideoxynucleosides, particularly ddC, may cause a dose related toxic neuropathy.[60] Information about HIV associated neuropathy is mainly derived from case reports and follow up, often incomplete, of clinic based case series. The reported frequency of occurrence of peripheral neuropathy varies considerably, which probably reflects differences in duration of infection among cases in the different series.

A distal, symmetric, painful, predominantly sensory axonal neuropathy is the commonest peripheral nerve syndrome associated with HIV infection.[61] Two large studies have shown that it is rare in the early stages of infection. In a cohort of around 800 HIV positive airforce personnel, all of whom had recently been considered fit for active duty, only 12 had symptoms or signs of neuropathy.[62] This finding confirmed the results of the multicentre AIDS cohort study.[63] Studies of groups of patients with more advanced disease have found higher rates.[60] Among 54 HIV infected patients referred to a neurological clinic over a 15 month period, distal symmetric peripheral neuropathies were present in 38. Two thirds of these had a distinct clinical syndrome characterised by painful paraesthesiae or sensations of burning in both feet and, in the eight patients who underwent sural nerve biopsy, axonal atrophy. There was a clear temporal relation between the onset of symptoms and cytomegalovirus infection. Neuropathies in the other patients were more heterogeneous. They included multiple mononeuropathy, isolated mono-neuropathies, and lumbosacral polyradiculopathy.

Demyelinating inflammatory polyneuropathy has been reported to occur at the time of seroconversion but it seems to be a rare event and is usually followed by complete recovery.[64]

Leprosy

In global terms leprosy remains an important cause of peripheral neuropathy. Fortunately, multidrug treatment and World Health Organisation surveillance programmes are having a major impact. Between 1990 and 1994 there was a 55% fall in the worldwide prevalence although part of the decrease may be due to changes in case definition. The highest prevalence of leprosy is in South East Asia (116 per 100 000) compared with 53 per 100 000 in Africa and 46 per 100 000 in Central and South America.[65] In Europe and North America the disease is only seen in immigrants.

Paraproteinaemic neuropathy

Serum monoclonal paraproteins were found in 10% of patients with otherwise unexplained peripheral neuropathy,[66] 10 times more often than expected in a population of elderly people. The associated paraproteins belonged to the IgM class in 60% of cases of neuropathy in two large series,[67 68] whereas in studies of serum paraproteins not associated with neuropathy, the IgG class accounted for 61% and IgM for only 8%.[69] The associated paraprotein is usually classified as being due to a monoclonal gammopathy of undetermined importance. This periphrasis implies absence of current malignancy but a potential for malignant transformation which requires follow up. Recognition of the association between the IgM paraprotein and demyelinating neuropathy led directly to the discovery of complement fixing antibodies directed against carbohydrate epitopes shared by myelin associated glycoprotein and a previously undiscovered peripheral nerve myelin glycolipid, sulphate-3-glucuronyl paragloboside. Transfer of the serum from patients with these antibodies has induced experimental demyelinating neuropathy in animals and there are anecdotal reports of improvement after treatment with plasma exchange and immunosuppression.[70] The antigenic targets of the antibody action of other paraproteins are gradually being defined, including IgM antibodies directed against ganglioside GM1 in multifocal motor neuropathy,[71] and IgM antibodies directed against disialosyl groups present on ganglioside GD3, GD1b, GT1b, and GQ1b in chronic large fibre sensory neuropathy.[72] The discovery of these autoantibodies in paraproteinaemic neuropathy has led to a search, which has sometimes been rewarding, for similar antibodies in peripheral neuropathy in which there is no paraprotein association. It is likely that other antibody specificities remain to be discovered. However, there are also other explanations for the association between a paraprotein and neuropathy including amyloid, vasculitis, and coincidence. Peripheral neuropathy is sometimes a feature of multiple myeloma, and is often present in the rarer cases of solitary myeloma.

Paraneoplastic neuropathy

Few studies have directly investigated how commonly neoplasms cause peripheral neuropathy. Lin et al[73] found that 2·3% of 520 cases of peripheral neuropathy attending neurological centres in Taiwan were due to neoplasm. Conversely between 2·5 and 5·5% of patients with lung or breast cancer have clinical evidence of a peripheral neuropathy.[74] Focal or multifocal radiculopathies, plexopathies, and neuropathies are usually due to infiltration or compression by the tumour. When symmetric polyneuropathies or neuronopathies are associated with a tumour, they are usually paraneoplastic manifestations. Paraneoplastic sensorimotor neuropathies are the most frequent syndrome, and are due to a wide variety of tumours, but especially carcinoma of the lung. Subacute sensory neuronopathy is a rather characteristic paraneoplastic syndrome, as about 20% of such cases do have an underlying carcinoma, which is usually a small cell lung carcinoma. In most cases investigation has disclosed the presence of antineuronal antibodies reacting with a family of nucleoproteins termed Hu, which strongly suggest an autoimmune pathogenesis.[75]

Toxic neuropathies

The peripheral nervous system is vulnerable to many toxic agents. In the past, heavy metals, especially lead, arsenic, and thallium, accounted for many cases of neuropathy. Occupational exposure to solvents such as n-hexane, carbon disulphide, and methyl-n-butyl ketone was previously a cause of peripheral sensorimotor neuropathy but now, in the western world at least, industrial legislation has resulted in strict control of permitted concentrations of these solvents in the workplace. Occasional outbreaks of neuropathy caused by industrial exposure are reported in economically developing countries. The epidemic of Jamaica ginger paralysis that occurred in the United States in 1930 and 1931 was due to the contamination of illicit alcohol with tri-*o*-cresyl phosphate. The story is an interesting one—not least because of the scale of the outbreak. It is estimated that 50 000 people were affected.[76] Other sudden outbreaks of peripheral neuropathy due to tri-*o*-cresyl phosphate have been reported in India, South Africa, and Morocco.[77-79]

More recently, an epidemic of a neurological syndrome the clinical features of which were dominated by a peripheral sensorimotor neuropathy, occurred in Spain as a result of the use of denatured rape seed oil that was sold as cooking oil. Neuropathological studies showed the unusual appearance of an intense inflammatory perineuritis followed by perineurial fibrosis with degeneration of myelinated axons. The oil contained high concentrations of peroxides and it was conjectured that nerve damage was caused by the action of free radicals.[80]

Alcohol

Peripheral nerve dysfunction is common in people who chronically misuse alcohol. There has been a long debate about whether this is due to a direct toxic effect of alcohol or whether it is a result of chronic nutritional deficiency. In a recent series of 107 alcoholic patients presenting at a Spanish hospital clinic, about a quarter showed abnormalities on tests of cardiovascular autonomic reflexes and a third fulfilled electrophysiological criteria of peripheral neuropathy.[81] Correlations between total lifetime dose of alcohol and sensory nerve compound action potential amplitudes were found but there was no relation to age, nutritional status, or the presence of other alcohol related diseases. Although thiamine deficiency has traditionally been thought to play a part in the pathogenesis of alcoholic neuropathy, a recent study of blood concentrations of free thiamine in chronic alcoholics showed no differences between those with and without peripheral neuropathy or between alcoholics and a control group.[82]

Bell's palsy

Bell's palsy, a unilateral, lower motor neuron facial paralysis, is the commonest condition affecting the facial nerve. Studies of incidence have been carried out in the United States and in Japan.[83-85] All relied on retrospective examination of hospital and clinic records to ascertain cases and are likely to have under-estimated the frequency of mild cases that remained undiagnosed or were treated in primary care. Crude incidence rates in these studies were fairly similar: in Rochester, Minnesota, USA, annual incidence was 25 per 100 000 population; in Laredo, Texas, USA, 23·5 per 100 000 in men and 32·7 per 100 000 in women; and in Ehime prefecture, Japan, 30 per 100 000 population. Rates for men and women were similar in Rochester and in the Ehime prefecture. Logistic regression analysis of the data from Rochester suggested that complete facial weakness, pain other than in or around the ear, and systemic hypertension were the most important predictors of incomplete recovery but out of 206 patients only 28 (14%) experienced incomplete recovery.

Evidence implicating local reactivation of herpes simplex virus type 1 in the aetiology of Bell's palsy comes from a recent report of a small series of patients who had decompressive surgery of the facial nerve.[86] Fragments of DNA specific for herpes simplex virus were detected by Southern blot analysis in endoneurial fluid from the affected facial nerve or in tissue from biopsy of the posterior auricular muscle after amplification by polymerase chain reaction in 11 out of 14 patients. No such fragments were found in fluid or tissue from the control group which consisted of nine patients with Ramsay-Hunt syndrome and 12 patients with a mixture of other diagnoses.

Neuralgic amyotrophy

A population based study of neuralgic amyotrophy in Rochester, Minnesota identified 11 cases over a period of 12 years giving an overall annual incidence of 1·6 per 100 000 population.[87] Retrospective analysis of case series and case reports have suggested various antecedent events: several infectious illnesses, immunisations, surgery, intravenous drug misuse, intravenous administration of radiological contrast medium, trauma in areas of the body remote from the brachial plexus, and childbirth. Detailed electrophysiological investigation of a small case series showed various lesions of individual peripheral nerves or their branches sometimes occurring singly and sometimes in combination.[88] These authors hypothesised that the course of these nerves, especially their location across joints, selectively exposed them to mild focal trauma and rendered them more susceptible to the disease.

Some cases of neuralgic amyotrophy are familial. The condition is apparently inherited as an autosomal dominant trait and may be associated with mildly dysmorphic facial features. In linkage studies of two large pedigrees, the gene was mapped to the distal part of the long arm of chromosome 17.[89] However, the disorder is genetically, as well as clinically, distinct from mutation in the PMP22 gene associated with hereditary neuropathy with liability to pressure palsies.[90]

Carpal tunnel syndrome

Carpal tunnel syndrome, caused by compression of the median nerve where it passes under the transverse carpal ligament in the wrist, is a common diagnosis in neurology and rheumatology outpatient clinics but there is remarkably little information about the frequency of its occurrence in the population generally. In a population based study of its prevalence in The Netherlands, carpal tunnel syndrome had been previously diagnosed in 3·4% of women and was present, undiagnosed, in a further 5·8%.[91] By contrast, in men the overall prevalence was only 0·6%. The medical records linkage system at the Mayo clinic has been used to study the incidence of the condition. The crude annual incidence rate during the period 1961 to 1980 was 99 per 100 000. Age adjusted sex specific rates showed a female to male ratio of 3:1.[92] Incidence rates increased during each sequential five year period of the study, from 88 per 100 000 to 125 per 100 000 but it was thought that this increase was more likely to reflect better recognition of the condition than a true increase in the underlying incidence. Rates increased with age in men, but in women incidence peaked in the 45 to 54 age group.

Many risk factors for carpal tunnel syndrome have been identified. Associations with diabetes, hypothyroidism, rheumatoid arthritis, amyloidosis, pregnancy, and haemodialysis have been found in retrospective studies of clinic based case series. Most cases associated with pregnancy resolve spontaneously after delivery.[93] Case-control studies have added other risk factors to the list including a history of gynaecological surgery, particularly hysterectomy and oophorectomy,[94] recent weight gain, and use of oestrogen replacement therapy.[95] Several studies have confirmed carpal tunnel syndrome as an occupational disease. Repetitive movements of the wrist, especially if they involve flexion or strong force, and the use of vibrating hand tools, are associated with a greatly increased risk. The economic consequences may not have been sufficiently recognised. Although follow up of case series suggests that treatment of carpal tunnel syndrome by surgical decompression is moderately effective in relieving pain, a study in the United States of 191 men and women of working age treated surgically found that the mean time lost from work was four months and that 8% of cases lost more than one year from work.[96]

In a large cohort of women followed up in the Oxford Family Planning Association contraceptive study, carpal tunnel syndrome was associated with obesity and a history of menstrual disorders. There was also a strong and unexpected association with smoking. Standardised first referral rates for carpal tunnel syndrome tripled as smoking increased from 0 to 25 or more cigarettes per day.[97]

Cervical radiculopathy

Cervical radiculopathy is another disorder of the peripheral nervous system that is common in clinical neurological practice but which has hardly been studied epidemiologically. The best information again comes from the Mayo clinic's medical record linkage system. Between 1976 and 1990, 561 patients from the population of Rochester and Olmsted county were diagnosed as having cervical radiculopathy. The overall annual incidence was 83 per 100 000 and rates were higher in men than in women.[98] Incidence was highest in the age group 50 to 54 years. The C6 or C7 nerve roots were affected in 64% of cases. Although recurrence of symptoms was common—32% of patients reported recurrence during a median time of follow up of five years—90% had few or no symptoms at their last follow up. Although population based, case finding in this study depended on medical records and it is almost certain that mild cases of the condition were underrepresented.

Conclusions

Except in the areas of diabetic neuropathy and Guillain-Barré syndrome, there have been disappointingly few sound epidemiological investigations of peripheral neuropathies. As a result, we know little about variations in the geographical distribution of even the common forms of neuropathy and almost nothing about trends in their incidence over time. There seem to be many opportunities for useful collaboration between neurologists and epidemiologists both in extending our knowledge of the descriptive epidemiology of peripheral neuropathies and in investigating aetiology. The methodology of case-control studies has been used successfully in identifying some of the antecedent infections associated with Guillain-Barré syndrome but has been underemployed in the investigation of other peripheral neuropathies. Although there have been large advances in understanding the genetics of hereditary neuropathies, the enormous variability of phenotypic expression of many of these mutations remains a puzzle. It has been suggested that interactions with environmental factors or between the gene and other genes may be important. If the first is correct, an epidemiological approach has the potential to increase our knowledge of both aetiology and pathogenesis.

1 Beghi E, Monticelli ML, Amoruso L, *et al*. Chronic symmetrical polyneuropathy in the elderly—a field screening investigation in 2 Italian regions 1. Prevalence and general characteristics of the sample. *Neurology* 1995;**45**:1832–6.
2 Bharucha NE, Bharucha AE, Bharucha EP. Prevalence of peripheral neuropathy in the Parsi community of Bombay. *Neurology* 1991;**41**:1315–7.

3 Savettieri G, Rocca WA, Salemi G, et al. Prevalence of diabetic neuropathy with somatic symptoms: a door-to-door survey in two Sicilian municipalities. *Neurology* 1993;43:1115–20.

4 Palumbo PJ, Elvehack LR, Whisnant JP. Neurological complications of diabetes mellitus: transient ischaemic attack, stroke and peripheral neuropathy. In: Schoenberg BS, ed. *Neurological epidemiology: principles and clinical applications.* New York: Raven Press, 1978:593–601.

5 Maser RE, Steenkiste AR, Dorman JS, et al. Epidemiological correlates of diabetic neuropathy: report from Pittsburgh Epidemiology of Diabetes Complications Study. *Diabetes* 1989;38:1456–61.

6 Franklin GM, Kahn LB, Baxter J, Marshall JA, Hamman RF. Sensory neuropathy in non-insulin-dependent diabetes mellitus: the San Luis Valley Diabetes Study. *Am J Epidemiol* 1990;131:633–43.

7 Partanen J, Niskanen L, Lehtinen J, Mervaala E, Siitonen O, Uusitupa M. Natural history of peripheral neuropathy in patients with non-insulin-dependent diabetes mellitus. *N Engl J Med* 1995;333:89–94.

8 Orchard TJ, Dorman JS, Maser RE, et al. Prevalence of complications in IDDM by sex and duration. Pittsburgh Epidemiology of Diabetes Complications Study II. *Diabetes* 1990;39:1116–24.

9 DCCT Research Group. The effect of intensive diabetes therapy on the development and progression of neuropathy. *Ann Intern Med* 1995;122:561–8.

10 Albers JW, Kenny DJ, Brown M, et al. Effect of intensive diabetes treatment on nerve conduction in the diabetes control and complications trial. *Ann Neurol* 1995;38:869–80.

11 Neil HA, Thompson AV, John S, McCarthy ST, Mann JI. Diabetic autonomic neuropathy: the prevalence of impaired heart rate variability in a geographically defined population. *Diabet Med* 1989;6:20–4.

12 Ewing DJ, Campbell IW, Clarke BF. The natural history of diabetic autonomic neuropathy. *Q J Med* 1980;49:95–108.

13 Flynn MD, O'Brien IA, Corrall RJM. The prevalence of autonomic and peripheral neuropathy in insulin-treated diabetic subjects. *Diabet Med* 1995;12:310–3.

14 Fleckenstein JF, Frank SM, Thuluvath PJ. Presence of autonomic neuropathy is a poor prognostic indicator in patients with advanced liver disease. *Hepatology* 1996;23:471–5.

15 Radhakrishnan K, El Mangoush MA, Gerryo SE. Descriptive epidemiology of selected neuromuscular disorders in Benghazi, Libya. *Acta Neurol Scand* 1987;75:95–100.

16 Osuntokun BO, Adeuja AOG, Schoenberg BS, et al. Neurological disorders in Nigerian Africans: a community-based study. *Acta Neurol Scand* 1987;75:13–21.

17 MacMillan JC, Harper PS. The Charcot-Marie-Tooth syndrome: clinical aspects from a population study in South Wales, UK. *Clinical Genetics* 1994;45:128–34.

18 Hagberg B, Westerberg B. Hereditary motor and sensory neuropathies in Swedish children. I. Prevalence and distribution by disability groups. *Acta Paediatrica Scandinavica* 1983;72:379–83.

19 Holmberg BH. Charcot-Marie-Tooth disease in northern Sweden: an epidemiological and clinical study. *Acta Neurol Scand* 1993;87:416–22.

20 Combarros O, Calleja J, Polo JM, Berciano J. Prevalence of hereditary motor and sensory neuropathy in Cantabria. *Acta Neurol Scand* 1987;75:9–12.

21 Skre H. Genetic and clinical aspects of Charcot-Marie-Tooth disease. *Clin Genet* 1974;6:98–118.

22 Nelis E, van Broeckhoven C. Estimation of the mutation frequencies in Charcot-Marie-Tooth disease type 1 and hereditary neuropathy with liability to pressure palsies: a European collaborative study. *Eur J Hum Genet* 1996;4: 25–33.

23 Blair IP, Nash J, Gordon MJ, Nicholson GA. Prevalence and origin of de novo duplications in Charcot-Marie-Tooth disease type 1A: first report of a de novo duplication with a maternal origin. *Am J Hum Genet* 1996;**58**:472–6.

24 Holmberg BH, Holmgren G, Nelis E, van Broeckhoven C, Westerberg B. Charcot-Marie-Tooth disease in northern Sweden: pedigree analysis and the presence of the duplication in chromosome 17p11·2. *J Med Genet* 1994;**31**:435–41.

25 Reilly M, Staunton H. Peripheral nerve amyloidosis. *Brain Pathol* 1996; **6**:163–77.

26 Hughes RAC, Rees JH. Clinical and epidemiological features of Guillain-Barré syndrome. *J Infections Dis* 1997.

27 Beghi E, Kurland LT, Mulder DW, Wiederholt WC. Guillain-Barré syndrome: clinicoepidemologic features and effect of influenza vaccine. *Arch Neurol* 1996;**42**:1053–7.

28 Govoni V, Granieri E, Casetta I, *et al.* The incidence of Guillain-Barré syndrome in Ferrara, Italy: is the disease really increasing? *J Neurol Sci* 1996;**137**:62–8.

29 Rees JH, Thompson RD, Hughes RAC. An epidemiological study of Guillain-Barré syndrome. *J Neurol Neurosurg Psychiatry* 1996;**61**:215.

30 Asbury AK, Cornblath DR. Assessment of current diagnostic criteria for Guillain-Barré syndrome. *Ann Neurol* 1990;**27**(suppl):S21–4.

31 Rees JH, Soudain SE, Gregson NA, Hughes RAC. A prospective case control study to investigate the relationship between Campylobacter jejuni infection and Guillain-Barré syndrome. *N Engl J Med* 1995;**333**:1374–9.

32 Kaplan JE, Katona P, Hurwitz ES, Schonberger LB. Guillain-Barré syndrome in the United States, 1979–80 and 1980–1. Lack of an association with influenza vaccination. *JAMA* 1982;**248**:698–700.

33 Kaplan JE, Schonberger LB, Hurwitz ES, Katona P. Guillain-Barré syndrome in the United States 1978–81; additional observations from the national surveillance system. *Neurology* 1983;**33**:633–7.

34 Barna M, Komatsu T, Zhengbiao B, Reiss CS. Sex differences in susceptibility to viral infection of the central nervous system. *J Neuroimmunol* 1996;**67**:31–9.

35 Roman GC. Tropical neuropathies. In: Hartung H-P, ed. *Peripheral neuropathies: part 1.* London: Baillière Tindall 1995;469–87.

36 Khoury SA. Guillain-Barré syndrome: epidemiology of an outbreak. *Am J Epidemiol* 1978;**197**:433–8.

37 McKhann GM, Cornblath DR, Griffin JW, *et al.* Acute motor axonal neuropathy: a frequent cause of acute flaccid paralysis in China. *Ann Neurol* 1993;**33**:333–42.

38 Ho TW, Mishu B, Li CY, *et al.* Guillain-Barré syndrome in northern China. Relationship to Campylobacter jejuni infection and anti-glycolipid antibodies. *Brain* 1995;**118**:597–605.

39 Winer JB, Hughes RAC, Anderson MJ, Jones DM, Kangro H, Watkins RFP. A prospective study of acute idiopathic neuropathy. II. Antecedent events. *J Neurol Neurosurg Psychiatry* 1988;**51**:613–8.

40 Van der Meché FGA, Schmitz PIM, Dutch Guillain-Barré Study Group. A randomized trial comparing intravenous immune globulin and plasma exchange in Guillain-Barré syndrome. *N Engl J Med* 1992;**326**:1123–9.

41 Mishu B, Ilyas A, Koski C, *et al.* Serologic evidence of previous Campylobacter jejuni infection in patients with Guillain-Barré syndrome. *Ann Intern Med* 1993;**118**:947–53.

42 Aspinall GO, Fujimoto S, McDonald AG, Pang H, Kurjanczyk LA, Penner JL. Lipopolysaccharides from *Campylobacter jejuni* associated with Guillain-Barré syndrome patients mimic human gangliosides in structure. *Infect Immun* 1994;**62**:2122–5.

43 Yuki N, Taki T, Takahashi M, *et al*. Penner's serotype 4 of Campylobacter jejuni has a lipopolysaccharide that bears a GM1 ganglioside epitope as well as one that bears a GD1a epitope. *Infect Immun* 1994;**62**:2101–3.

44 Gregson NA, Rees JH, Hughes RAC. Reactivity between IgG antiGM1 ganglioside antibodies and the lipopolysaccharide fractions of Campylobacter jejuni isolates from patients with Guillain-Barré syndrome. *J Neuroimmunol* 1997;**73**:28–36..

45 Li C, Xue P, Tian W, Liu R, Yang C. Experimental Campylobacter jejuni infection in the chicken: an animal model of axonal Guillain-Barré syndrome. *J Neurol Neurosurg Psychiatry* 1996;**61**:279–84.

46 Illa I, Ortiz N, Gallard E, Juarez C, Grau JM, Dalakas MC. Acute axonal Guillain-Barré syndrome with IgG antibodies against motor axons following parenteral gangliosides. *Ann Neurol* 1995;**38**:218–24.

47 Landi G, D'Alessandro R, Dossi BC, Ricci SSi. Gangliosides and the Guillain-Barré syndrome. *BMJ* 1994;**308**:1638.

48 Landi G, D'Alessandro R, Dossi BC, Ricci S, Simone IL, Ciccone A. Guillain-Barré syndrome after exogenous gangliosides in Italy. *BMJ* 1993;**307**:1463–4.

49 Beghi E. Exposure to exogenous gangliosides and Guillain-Barré syndrome. *Neuroepidemiology* 1995;**14**:45–8.

50 Hughes RAC. *Guillain-Barré syndrome*. Heidelberg: Springer-Verlag, 1990.

51 Schonberger LB, Bregman DJ, Sullivan-Bolynai JZ, *et al*. Guillain-Barre syndrome following vaccination in the national influenza immunization program, United States 1976–7. *Am J Epidemiol* 1979;**110**:105–23.

52 Hughes RAC, Rees J, Smeeton N, Winer J. Vaccines and Guillain-Barré syndrome. *BMJ* 1996;**312**:1475–6.

53 Winer JB, Hughes RAC, Osmond C. A prospective study of acute idiopathic neuropathy. I. Clinical features and their prognostic value. *J Neurol Neurosurg Psychiatry* 1988;**51**:605–12.

54 McKhann GM, Griffin JW, Cornblath DR, *et al*. Plasmapheresis and Guillain-Barré syndrome: analysis of prognostic factors and the effect of plasmapheresis. *Ann Neurol* 1988;**23**:347–53.

55 Gibbels E, Giebisch U. Natural course of acute and chronic monophasic inflammatory demyelinating polyneuropathies (IDP). *Acta Neurol Scand* 1992;**85**:282–91.

56 Hughes R, Sanders E, Hall S, Atkinson P, Colchester A, Payan J. Subacute idiopathic demyelinating polyradiculoneuropathy. *Arch Neurol* 1992;**49**:612–6.

57 McCombe PA, Pollard JD, McLeod JG. Chronic inflammatory demyelinating polyradiculoneuropathy. *Brain* 1987;**110**:1617–30.

58 Mélendez-Vásquez C, Redford J, Choudhary PP, *et al*. Immunological investigation of chronic inflammatory demyelinating polyradiculoneuropathy. *J Neuroimmunol* 1997;**73**:124–34.

59 Hughes RAC, Choudhary PP, Osborn M, Rees JH, Sanders EACM. Immunisation and risk of relapse of Guillain-Barré syndrome or chronic inflammatory demyelinating polyradiculoneuropathy. *Muscle Nerve* 1996;**19**:1230–1.

60 Fichtenbaum CJ, Clifford DB, Powderly WG. Risk factors for dideonucleoside-induced toxic neuropathy in patients with the human immunodeficiency virus infection. *J Acquir Immune Defic Syndr Hum Retrovirol* 1995;**10**:169–74.

61 Fuller GN, Jacobs JN, Guiloff RJ. Nature and incidence of peripheral nerve syndromes in HIV infection. *J Neurol Neurosurg Psychiatry* 1993;**56**:372–81.

62 Barohn RJ, Gronseth GS, LeForce BR, *et al*. Peripheral nervous system involvement in a large cohort of human immunodeficiency virus-infected individuals. *Arch Neurol* 1993;**50**:167–71.

63 McArthur JC, Cohen BA, Selnes OA, *et al*. Low prevalence of neurological and neuropsychological abnormalities in otherwise healthy HIV-1 infected individuals: results from the multicenter AIDS cohort study. *Ann Neurol* 1989;**26**:601–11.

64 Leger JM, Bouche P, Bolgert F, *et al*. The spectrum of polyneuropathies in patients infected with HIV. *J Neurol Neurosurg Psychiatry* 1989;**52**:1369–74.

65 World Health Organisation. Progress towards eliminating leprosy as a public health problem. *Wkl Epidemiol Rec* 1994;**20**:145–51.

66 Kelly JJ, Kyle RA, O'Brien PC, Dyck PJ. The prevalence of monoclonal gammopathy in peripheral neuropathy. *Neurology* 1981;**31**:1480–3.

67 Yeung KB, Thomas PK, King RHM, *et al*. The clinical spectrum of peripheral neuropathies associated with benign monoclonal IgM, IgG, and IgA paraproteinaemia. Comparative clinical, immunological, and nerve biopsy findings. *J Neurol* 1991;**238**:383–91.

68 Gosselin S, Kyle RA, Dyck PJ. Neuropathy associated with monoclonal gammopathies of undetermined significance. *Ann Neurol* 1991;**30**:54–61.

69 Axelsson U, Bachmann R, Hällén J. Frequency of pathological proteins (M components) in 6995 sera from an adult population. *Acta Med Scand* 1966;**179**:235–47.

70 Tatum AH. Experimental paraprotein neuropathy, demyelination by passive transfer of human IgM anti-myelin-associated glycoprotein. *Ann Neurol* 1993;**33**:502–6.

71 Nobile-Orazio E. Multifocal motor neuropathy. *J Neurol Neurosurg Psychiatry* 1996;**60**:599–603.

72 Willison HJ, Paterson G, Veitch J, Inglis G, Barnett SC. Peripheral neuropathy associated with monoclonal IgM anti-Pr$_2$ cold agglutinins. *J Neurol Neurosurg Psychiatry* 1993;**56**:1178–83.

73 Lin KP, Kwan SY, Chen SY, *et al*. Generalized neuropathy in Taiwan: an etiologic survey. *Neuroepidemiology* 1993;**12**:257–61.

74 Croft PB, Wilkinson M. The incidence of carcinomatous neuromyopathy in patients with various types of carcinoma. *Brain* 1965;**88**:427–34.

75 Smitt PS, Posner JB. Paraneoplastic peripheral neuropathy. In: Hartung H-P, ed. *Peripheral neuropathies: part I*. London: Baillière Tindall, 1996:443–68.

76 Morgan JP, The Jamaica ginger paralysis. *JAMA* 1982;**248**:1864–7.

77 Vora DD, Dastur DK, Beatriz M, *et al*. Toxic polyneuropathies in Bombay due to ortho-cresyl phosphate poisoning. *J Neurol Neurosurg Psychiatry* 1962;**25**:234–42.

78 Susser M, Stein Z. An outbreak of tri-ortho-cresyl phosphate poisoning in Durban. *Br J Ind Med* 1957;**14**:111.

79 Smith HV Spalding JMK. Outbreak of paralysis in Morocco due to ortho-cresyl phosphate poisoning. *Lancet* 1959;**ii**:1019.

80 Ricoy JR, Cabello A, Rodriguez J, Tellez I. Neuropathological studies on the toxic syndrome related to adulterated rapeseed oil in Spain. *Brain* 1983; **106**:817–35.

81 Monforte R, Estruch R, VallsSole J, Nicholas J, Urbano Marquez A. Autonomic and peripheral neuropathies in patients with chronic alcoholism: a dose-related toxic effect of alcohol. *Arch Neurol* 1995;**52**:45–51.

82 Poupon RE, Gervaise G, Riant P, Houin G, Tillement JP. Blood thiamine and thiamine phosphate concentrations in excessive drinkers with or without peripheral neuropathy. *Alcohol Alcohol* 1990;**25**:605–11.

83 Katusic SK, Beard CM, Wiederholt WC, *et al*. Incidence, clinical features, and prognosis in Bell's palsy, Rochester, Minnesota, 1968–82. *Ann Neurol* 1986;**20**:622–7.

84 Yanagihara N. Incidence of Bell's palsy. *Ann Otol Rhinol Laryngol* 1988;**97**:3–4.

85 Brandenburg NA, Annegers JF. Incidence and risk factors for Bell's palsy in Laredo, Texas: 1974–82 *Neuroepidemiology* 1993;**12**:313–25.

86 Murakami S, Mizobuchi M, Nakashiro Y, Doi T, Hato N, Yanagihara N. Bell's palsy and herpes simplex virus: identification of viral DNA in endoneurial fluid and muscle. *Ann Intern Med* 1996;**124**:27–30.

87 Beghi E, Kurland LT, Mulder DW, Nicolosi A. Brachial plexus neuropathy in the population of Rochester, Minnesota, 1970–81. *Ann Neurol* 1985;**18**:320–3.

88 England JD, Sumner AJ. Neuralgic amyotrophy: an increasingly diverse entity. *Muscle Nerve* 1987;**10**:60–8.

89 Pellegrino JE, Rebbeck TR, Brown MJ, Bird TD, Chance PF. Mapping of hereditary neuralgic amyotrophy (familial brachial plexus neuropathy) to distal chromosome 17q. *Neurology* 1996;**46**:1128–32.

90 Gouider R, LeGuern E, Emile J, *et al.* Hereditary neuralgic amyotrophy and hereditary neuropathy with liability to pressure palsies. *Neurology* 1994;**44**:2250–2.

91 DeKrom MC, Knipschild PG, Kester AD, Thijs CT, Boekkooi, PF, Spaans F. Carpal tunnel syndrome: prevalence in the general population. *J Clin Epidemiol* 1992;**45**:373–6.

92 Stevens JC, Sun S, Beard CM, O'Fallon WM, Kurland LT. Carpal tunnel syndrome in Rochester, Minnesota, 1961–80. *Neurology* 1988;**38**:134–8.

93 Ekman-Ordeberg G, Salgeback S, Ordeberg G. Carpal tunnel syndrome in pregnancy. A prospective study. *Acta Obstet Gynecol Scand* 1987;**66**:233–5.

94 Cannon LJ, Bernacki EJ, Walter SD. Personal and occupational factors associated with carpal tunnel syndrome. *J Occup Med* 1981;**23**:255–8.

95 Dieck GS, Kelsey JL. An epidemiologic study of the carpal tunnel syndrome in an adult female population. *Prev Med* 1985;**14**:63–9.

96 Adams ML, Franklin GM, Barnhart S. Outcome of carpal tunnel surgery in Washington State workers' compensation. *Am J Ind Med* 1994;**25**:527–36.

97 Vessey MP, Villard-Mackintosh L, Yeates D. Epidemiology of carpal tunnel syndrome in women of child-bearing age. Findings in a large cohort study. *Int J Epidemiol* 1990;**19**:43–7.

98 Radhakrishnan K, Litchy WJ, O'Fallon WM, Kurland LT. Epidemiology of cervical radiculopathy: a population based study from Rochester, Minnesota. *Brain* 1994;**117**:325–35.

6 Neurological disability

DERICK WADE

> - A disabling neurological illness can be considered at one or more of four levels. The four levels are the organ (pathology), the person (impairment), behaviour (disability) and performance in a social role (handicap).
> - The extent of problems at one level does not necessarily predict the extent at another level.
> - External factors tend to have a greater influence on how disability determines handicap than on how pathology or impairment determine disability.
> - Research is needed to investigate relations between the different levels and the factors that influence them.

Epidemiological research aims to establish the causes, mechanisms, and natural history of illness. It has traditionally focused on specific diseases, using data obtained from populations to investigate the factors related to the disease of interest. The relevant data will usually include some of the characteristics of the patient; the manifestation of the disease; the patient's history and social status; the patient's past and present environment; and the characteristics of other people without the disease. Analysis aims to establish the nature and strength of the interrelations between these factors and the occurrence of disease. In this way epidemiology has answered questions such as: Why does this disease occur? What causes it? What is likely to happen? How can we prevent disease or improve recovery?

Often epidemiological research will incidentally also answer the question, How common is this disease? Consequently a second, much more recent focus has been the use of epidemiological data on the frequency (incidence or prevalence) of diseases to plan the delivery of health services. This secondary analysis has tried to answer the questions: How many people will develop or have the disease? What services may be needed by patients with this disease? However, most of the data used come from studies designed to disentangle the causes or natural history of disease. Very few studies have set out to determine the need of the community for specific health services, not least because it is difficult to determine a patient's need for an intervention (defined as their ability to benefit from the intervention) from the information available.

More broadly, epidemiological research also "strives to develop a theoretical framework for the understanding of health experience".[1] Disability is, for many people with neurological disease, an integral if not overwhelming part of their health experience. Therefore this review starts with a consideration of disease based epidemiology; the frequency of neurological disability; and the need for services. However, the information available relating to these topics is too poor to allow specific conclusions, and the bulk of this review considers a theoretical framework of illness, the predictions this theory makes, and some of the available evidence relating to these predictions.

Frequency of neurological disability

For disabling neurological disease, there is currently a major focus on planning appropriate services especially for common chronic diseases and their rehabilitation. This topic was reviewed 10 years ago,[2] and epidemiological studies have been reviewed since in relation to various specific services.[3-7] There are several problems with using currently available epidemiological data to plan services and to estimate disability.

The first problem with using currently available disease based epidemiological studies is that patients with rare diseases such as tuberous sclerosis will often not have their problems specifically accounted for.[8] Although each individual disease is rare, it is likely that the combined incidence and, more importantly, prevalence of these rare diseases is sufficient to make a major impact on health services. Furthermore, the epidemiology of many rare diseases is poorly researched.

Next, this disease based approach does not account for services needed for people presenting to medical services with a symptom for diagnosis. For example, the number of patients referred with "possible multiple sclerosis" probably exceeds the true incidence of multiple sclerosis by a factor of five. Although this has not been formally researched, data from routine clinical practice highlights the number of patients who have no clear-cut diagnosis.[9 10] None the less, patients with diagnostically uncertain problems, such as undiagnosed tremor, may be disabled and need disability services.[11]

Thirdly, using data on the epidemiology of the disease itself to study the epidemiology of (neurologically based) disability assumes reasonable information about the proportion of incident or prevalent cases who are in fact disabled (if disability is the interest) or who might benefit from services (if service planning is the interest). Such information is rarely, if ever, available. Establishing need, the ability to benefit from an intervention, is particularly difficult because: (a) there is limited evidence concerning the ability to benefit; and (b) this requires an assessment by an experienced clinician.

Lastly, secondary analysis of epidemiological data does not easily allow calculation of the number of people needing a specific service such as advice on wheelchairs, or urodynamic investigations and advice on continence, or spasticity management. These important practical problems, which have important resource implications, arise as a relatively rare consequence of many separate diseases and have not been specifically studied.

Few if any studies have specifically focused on the nature or extent of disability within a specific disease, let alone specifically focusing on the incidence or prevalence of specific disabilities across several diseases. There are no useful studies allowing meaningful comparison of neurological disability between geographic areas, or over time, or between diseases.

Only one specific epidemiological point needs to be made in relation to neurological disability. Neurological disease or injury accounts for the vast majority of patients with severe disability.[12-17] Specialists with training in neurology and disability are obviously needed to help manage this large and important population of patients who have specific problems not seen in patients with non-neurological diseases.

Otherwise much of the information relating to the traditional epidemiology of neurological disease has been reviewed in this series. More importantly the gaps in available data mentioned above cannot be filled with much accuracy until more systematic studies focusing on disability are undertaken. Therefore this review will not attempt to calculate the incidence or prevalence of neurological disability because any conclusions will be too uncertain to be useful.

Instead this review will suggest to the reader that there is another important area awaiting epidemiological research. This area is analogous to the study of the causes of disease. It is the study of the mechanisms leading to disability, an area still awaiting appreciable systematic epidemiological research despite its recognition in the past.[1 18]

This review will argue that investigations into the relations between disability and other areas is urgently needed and that traditional methods of epidemiological research would be very appropriate to investigate the nature and genesis of disability. These methods could and should be used to increase our understanding of the questions: How and why do some people become disabled whereas others do not? How many people need disability services? What is the natural history of disability?

The review has several limitations. Formal searching of the medical literature has not been undertaken. Identifying appropriate studies is difficult, because abstracts and computer indexes do not mention the presence or otherwise of information on disability. Moreover, this review concerns a form of epidemiological research that is not yet specifically recognised. Next, I have a biased interest in neurological disability and believe that the subject is not given sufficient attention or resources. Consequently most of the studies referred to have been found in the pursuit of that interest; they have been selected because they relate to the hypotheses being put forward. There will be gaps and may be important omissions.

The review puts forward a thesis for debate and does not intend to prove the thesis absolutely. The thesis put forward is that the model of illness developed within the field of rehabilitation medicine should now be tested against empirical epidemiologically based data. The model makes certain predictions about the factors which may impact on disability and the relative importance of those factors. These predictions can be tested. This review will supply some relevant data but better studies are needed to consolidate and improve the model.

World Health Organisation Model of Impairment, Disability and Handicap, and terminology

The traditional epidemiological approach to disease both depended on and itself helped to develop a new model of illness. It drew attention to the importance of infectious agents, social factors, environmental poisons, etc in the genesis of disease. Before epidemiological research, disease was often mysterious and misunderstood. Unfortunately disability is still often misunderstood, and debates about the definitions of disability and rehabilitation can be endless, and often complicate and dominate discussion.

Therefore, before reviewing the relevant data, it is vital to have a clear understanding of the framework involved when discussing disability, and to agree the terminology. This review uses concepts and definitions which are commonly referred to as the World Health Organisation model of Impairment, Disability and Handicap (WHO ICIDH).[19-25] This model can be derived using a systems approach to analyse illness (defined here as the personal experience of disease), and it divides illness into four hierarchical levels (see table 6.1 and figure 6.1). The model has a long, largely unpublished history[18-21] and is still largely theoretical.[25] One vital role of future epidemiological research will be to validate this model, or to alter and improve it.

The terminology and definitions given in table 6.1 are not identical to those used in the official document.[19] They are sufficiently close to be acceptable but some points must be remembered. Firstly, it is probably best to conceive of or refer to "changes at the level of" handicap, rather than handicap (and similarly for the other levels). Next, there is no good word for normal except the absence of (for example) impairment. Thirdly, many people will use these words in other ways, usually in other contexts. The definitions given here are all referred to in the context of illness.

Table 6.1   The four levels of illness in the WHO ICIDH model

Word	Level/system affected	Definition	Synonym
Pathology	Organ or organ system	Any abnormality of macroscopic, microscopic, or biochemical structure or function affecting an organ or organ system	Diagnosis or disease
Impairment	Organism	Any abnormality of structure or function of, or affecting, the whole body independent of any specific environment	Symptoms and signs
Disability	Interaction between organism and environment (people and objects)—that is, behaviour	Any change or restriction in a patient's goal directed behaviour or behavioural repertoire, usually manifest as dependence	Functional limitations
Handicap	Meaning attached to behaviour by self and others	Any alteration in a patient's status (position) in society including alterations in roles	Social consequences

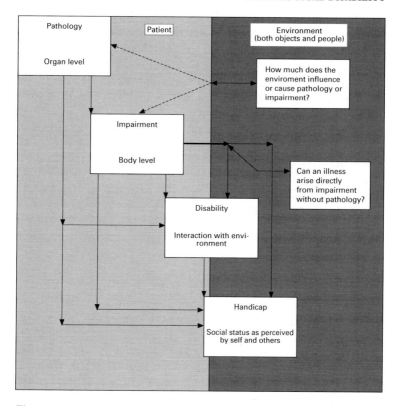

Figure 6.1   WHO ICIDH model of illness. Arrows on left refer to generally accepted relations. Arrows on right and dashed arrows are less generally accepted. Strength of relations unknown.

The WHO ICIDH model emphasises that disability is best considered as a change in or restriction on a person's behaviour.[22–24] Disability is not synonymous either with being in a wheelchair or with being dependent. Within this model rehabilitation is synonymous with "the management of neurological disability" and it can be defined as: "an educational, reiterative, problem solving process which focuses on disability and aims to maximise the patient's social role functioning and to minimise the somatic and emotional distress experienced by both patient and family." Within this definition it must be recognised that (*a*) one aim of rehabilitation is to minimise handicap, *not* to minimise disability and (*b*) that the other aims relate to stress and distress experienced by patients and families. The main objectives of rehabilitation for the patient are to maximise his or her

123

behavioural repertoire; to optimise the environment; and to help with emotional distress.

Epidemiological research is needed to consider several important questions. Are the concepts and definitions supported by the empirical data? What are the interrelations between the four levels?[25] How does distress of the family and patient relate to disability (or impairment)? What interventions are most likely to assist with the aims and objectives of rehabilitation? Some studies providing data relating to some of these questions will be reviewed.

Nature and genesis of disability

The WHO ICIDH model is based on the premise that four separate but related systems may be affected within any illness: the organ; the body (a collection of organs); the person interacting with the environment; and the person's position within their own social network. It was assumed within the original model that there is a relatively straight pathway from pathology through impairment to disability and on to handicap (arrows on the left in figure 6.1).[18-21] However, it was recognised that sometimes the chain of causation could jump one level. The possibility of jumping from pathology to handicap was not considered. The possibility that some illness may arise primarily at the level of impairment or even at the level of disability has also not been formally raised (see figure 6.1).

Epidemiological research could be used to investigate the nature and genesis of disability and handicap just as it has previously been used to investigate the nature and genesis of disease. In fact few studies have specifically investigated the links between pathology, impairment, disability, and handicap in a formal way. Most of the information available comes from studies which focused on other matters.

Pathology and impairment

The model predicts a relatively close relation between the impairments seen or experienced and the underlying pathological process, both in quality (that each pathological lesion will be associated with specific impairments) and in quantity (that more

124

severe disease will be associated with impairments of greater severity or more impairments). However, the model also predicts that pathology may occur without impairment and that impairment may possibly occur without pathology.

The traditional medical diagnostic approach depends on a relatively close qualitative link between impairments (symptoms and signs) and the underlying disease (pathological process). However, although the link between pathological process and impairment is relatively close and invaluable in making a diagnosis, it is not absolute. Examples of this weak link include patients without recorded symptoms found after death to have the pathological changes of multiple sclerosis; and the large size achieved by some malignant brain tumours before their clinical presentation.

The links between impairment and pathology are well documented and form the basis of all medicine. Qualitatively impairments can be used to allocate stroke patients into broad diagnostic groups locating the area of cerebral infarction.[26] Quantitatively there is a link between the volume of brain loss after stroke and acute impairments.[27] In multiple sclerosis relatively strong links have been found between total lesion load shown on MRI and the extent of cognitive impairment (Moller *et al*[28] and review by Rao[29]).

With more sensitive techniques for detecting pathology, the weaknesses in the links between pathological processes and impairments are becoming more apparent. It is now possible to detect the pathology of Huntington's chorea using genetic tests before any clinical manifestations are apparent.[30] The use of MRI to investigate patients with single symptomatic episodes of (for example) optic neuritis can demonstrate more widespread pathology.[31] Investigation of elderly people presenting with epilepsy will sometimes disclose silent cerebral infarction,[32] and clinically silent episodes of cerebral infarction are common.[33][34]

The relation between specific impairments and specific lesion location also needs much further research, and it is possible that many neurologists and psychologists place too much weight on the association between specific impairments and specific lesion locations. For example, it is common clinical practice in management of head injury to equate poor performance on the Wisconsin card sorting test (an impairment) with frontal lobe damage (a pathological lesion). The minimal evidence available suggests that there may be little or no linkage between poor performance on this test and specific locations of cerebral damage[35] (although there may be[36]). Similarly, it is difficult to determine any unique or central area of damage underlying aphasia.[37]

It may be concluded that some predictions are upheld: the qualitative and quantitative links between pathology and impairment are reasonable and pathology may occur without impairment. However, the strength of these links has not be studied closely in many situations, and caution is needed when attributing impairments to pathology demonstrated by modern sensitive investigations. More caution is needed when attributing specific impairments to specific lesion locations. Thus although general associations exist between impairments and lesion location, much further detailed research into the relation between pathology and impairment is needed, including studies of the strength of any associations between impairment and pathology (for example, their specificity and sensitivity). It would also be of interest to discover what factors affect the development of impairments with pathology; why are some large lesions asymptomatic?

Pathology and disability

The WHO ICIDH model predicts that the links between pathology and disability are not very close in either direction. In this context it is worth remembering that disability is manifest most obviously as dependence, and that providing care to alleviate dependence requires resources.

Despite this prediction, the current use of diagnosis related groups (DRGs) (healthcare resource groups, HRGs in Britain) as a means of defining resource groups is based, in part at least, on the untested assumption that the resources used by a patient are related to pathological diagnosis. In fact it is common experience that use of health resources is dominated by the need to provide care, not by treatments or investigations specific to the pathology. For this reason, if no other, there is an urgent need to investigate the relation between pathological diagnosis and disability. At present there are no studies comparing levels of disability between different diseases, and none explicitly comparing specific disabilities between diseases. Moreover, one study on selected inpatients has shown that health resources used by disabled people are not related to diagnosis.[38]

There are a few specific examples of pathology which are clearly and closely related to specific disabilities. The best example is spinal cord injury, in which the lesion and, more importantly, its location define quite repeatably the disabilities experienced. However, there are few other instances of such a close relation, and in most cases it is likely that the pattern and extent of disability is only weakly related, if at all, to diagnosis. Unless (or until) a close relation is shown between pathological diagnosis and resource use, it would be sensible to develop disability related groups as a means of justifying or giving resources.

The more interesting relation to investigate is that between the extent of pathology and the nature and extent of disability within a group of patients with the same diagnosis (pathologically homogenous). For many diseases, such as Parkinson's disease, it is not directly possible to quantify the extent of pathology in life. If it is assumed that pathology in Parkinson's disease increases with duration of disease then there may be a reasonable link between extent of pathology and level of disability, but this assumption may not be valid. In multiple sclerosis there are now several studies investigating the link between changes seen on MRI and disability.[39-41] Although the results are not all in agreement, it can be concluded that any link between the extent of multiple sclerosis pathology and disability is relatively weak. In stroke the few studies investigating the relation between CT changes and longer term levels of disability have found at best a weak link between the volume or location of a stroke and the resultant long term disability.[42 43]

At present the prediction of weak links if any between the type of pathological process (diagnosis) and associated disability is untested because the epidemiological evidence is almost non-existent. The very few studies of patients with a single diagnosis which provide data on the link between the extent of pathology and the level of disability support the hypothesis that there may be a weak statistical link in groups of patients, but in an individual patient the link is not clinically useful.

Impairment and disability

The model predicts a relatively close relation between impairment and disability, although this relation will be complicated by several other influences. Two are discussed below and the third, the environment, is discussed later.

The first complicating factor is that patients may learn to achieve their behavioural goals in other ways when an impairment is present. For example, someone can learn to write using their left hand if they lose their right hand; someone can learn to walk despite a stiff (or even absent) leg; aids, equipment and other environmental changes can allow someone to have more independent behaviours despite unchanging impairment; and new goals and behaviours may develop in place of old ones (for example, someone may develop new work skills or new hobbies). Therefore the relation between a specific impairment and a specific disability might vary both over time, as adaptation occurs, and between patients dependent on their motivation, adaptability, and opportunities. Only epidemiological research investigating large groups and collecting all relevant ancillary data can illuminate this problem successfully.

The second and even more important feature is that it is rare for a single impairment to be present on its own and it is unusual for a single impairment to be the only or major cause of a specific disability.[25] Normal behaviour depends on the integrated functioning of many skills. Disruption of one skill alone may sometimes lead directly to a single specific disability but this will be rare. More usually disruption of several skills will be needed to cause a disability. Indeed, sometimes the impairment might be compensated for under most conditions and disability will only be disclosed under stress. For example, it has been shown that standing balance using a prosthesis after amputation is made worse by a stressful cognitive task in the early stages of rehabilitation.[44] Thus a specific disability might arise in many ways from different combinations of many different impairments and, conversely, a single impairment may lead to or be an influence on several disabilities.[25]

To an extent this complexity has been shown by the multivariate prognostic equations developed (for example) in stroke research[45]; in most studies and equations there are two to four early impairments which relate to later disability. These studies have investigated the prognostic relation between current impairment and future disability. Concurrent comparisons are less common but do also show that several impairments relate to the level of disability.[46–53] Sometimes the combination of impairments will arise from several diseases (the essence of geriatric medicine).[54]

128

None the less, studies have found the expected relations between the presence or severity of a single impairment and the severity of disability. In the acute phase after stroke there is an unsurprising relation between the degree of motor loss and the extent of disability.[46] Other studies have shown the expected positive relations between strength of various leg muscles and gait speed[47 48] and between the degree of motor loss after stroke and arm function.[49] The specific impairment of tremor is associated with a higher level of dependence in activities of daily living (ADL).[11] Mobility disability in spinal cord injury is closely related to motor impairment.[55]

In relation to neurological disability, epidemiological studies disclose one important but often neglected fact: many patients with disabling neurological disease have considerable impairment of both cognitive skills and emotional control. Up to half of all patients with stroke have problems with memory and other cognitive skills[56 57]; up to half of all patients with multiple sclerosis have measurable cognitive losses[29]; cognitive losses occur in motor neuron disease, albeit at a relatively minor level,[58] and in at least 20% of patients with Parkinson's disease[59]; and they are an important feature in many other pathological states, such as Huntington's chorea, Friedreich's ataxia, muscular dystrophy, and (obviously) head injury. The frequency of changes in emotional control or state has been less well studied, but it is likely to be important in stroke,[60] multiple sclerosis,[61] motor neuron disease[58], head injury, and many other situations.

These epidemiological findings are important for two reasons. Rehabilitation is concerned with altering behaviour through learning and adaptation. This depends on the patient being able to learn, and it is often their very ability to learn and adapt that is compromised by the disabling disease. Moreover, most behaviour is goal directed, and changes in emotional state may have a major influence on behaviour and adaptability. There is minor, weak evidence that altering depression may reduce disability.[62 63]

Unfortunately many people have a very mechanistic view of disability and ignore or overlook the importance of these "hidden" impairments. For example, most service provision refers to patients with "physical disability". The more accurate phrase would be "patients with motor impairment" but this grouping ignores the reality that motor impairment is rarely the major factor causing disability.

It may be concluded that the evidence supports the general relations expected between impairment and disability. However, they are only apparent either when the level of impairment is extreme or in specific diseases. The importance of concurrent relations between impairment, especially combinations of impairment and disability, has yet to be explored in a systematic manner. Hopefully further epidemiological research will eventually convince service planners that emotional and cognitive impairments are central to understanding most disability and that "physical disability" does not exist.

Disability, handicap, and the environment

Because disability refers to the patient's interaction with his or her environment, this model predicts that environmental factors will have a significant influence on disability and an even greater influence on handicap. The extent of this influence on disability will be moderate, probably less than the influence of the patient's impairments. A patient's position in society is determined primarily by how other people interpret and perceive role performance and so this model predicts that handicap will be greatly influenced by a patient's social environment.

The presence of HIV infection gives an example of the importance of social factors in determining handicap, and it also shows that a pathological process can cause handicap directly. A person found on incidental testing to have HIV infection will not have any impairment or disability. However, once the fact of infection is known to others it will affect personal relations, housing, employment, etc. The handicap is determined by the attitude and perception of other people.

There are few studies appertaining to this area. Observational studies have suggested that people who live alone are more independent.[64] but it is uncertain whether this relation reflects selective loss from the study of more dependent people into institutional care or the effects of necessity. There are very few studies of the relation between environmental adaptations and disability, even at the level of simple aids such as ankle-foot orthoses.[65] It is worth noting that independence in some activities such as stair climbing may be important in a British context but of little importance in parts of the world such as Australia, where most accommodation is single storey.

Identifying the influences on handicap will be difficult, not least because the definition and measurement of handicap continues to be extremely difficult.[66] Moreover, it is likely that many influences will lie well outside the remit of health services. Consequently it is difficult to cite studies. One study has investigated the relation between one dimension of handicap and disability, finding (as predicted) that financial resources alleviate handicap.[67] Another study investigated the factors influencing handicap caused by vertigo.[68] This study, which is probably more accurately considered as a study of disability, started to disentangle the relations between symptoms (vertigo), other secondary impairments (fear, emotional distress), and restriction of activities. A study on the factors affecting social functioning after stroke also showed the complexity of interrelations between emotional state, age, intelligence, sex, and premorbid interests.[69]

Therefore the major conclusion to be drawn is that much further research is needed to provide data to allow the concept of handicap to be tested empirically; to determine the relation between a patient's behavioural repertoire and the level of handicap; to investigate the relation between specific disabilities and handicap in different cultures and societies; and to determine how other environmental factors relate to disability and handicap. For example, altering regulations related to disability allowances might reduce or increase handicap,[25] and empirical data would help guide decisions.

Illness without disease

Using a systems analytical approach to derive the WHO ICIDH model shows that not all illness has an underlying pathology. If the hypothesis is that the model encompasses four separate systems, then systems theory would predict that illness may emerge at any level without a specific abnormality at a lower level. In other words it is possible that not all "neurological disability" arises from neurological disease.

In fact this is a well recognised phenomenon. In our own local "young disabled unit" 5% to 10% of patients in wheelchairs do not have any diagnosed neurological (or specific psychiatric) disease (unpublished observations). More generally it is well reported that patients may present with neurological impairments and disability and yet have no demonstrable neurological pathology.[70]

Furthermore, it has long been recognised that external stress such as bereavement (a change in personal environment) is associated with increased mortality and that depression (an impairment) is associated with altered immunity (a pathological state).[71] Interactions between the nervous system and changes in the immune system have been reviewed recently.[72] Poverty is associated with a higher level of mortality,[73 74] again showing a possible link "in reverse" with factors at the level of handicap in some way causing pathological abnormalities (and hence death or later neurological disability).

Some specific common diagnoses may in fact represent illness arising at the level of impairment. Headache and the disability and handicap associated with it may well be the commonest example of an illness without a specific underlying pathology. Population based studies have generally failed to substantiate any specific types of headache[75 76] and it is possible that any reported biochemical or other changes at the level of pathology associated with migraine are simply epiphenomena, occurring as a result of the impairment. The development of frozen shoulder after myocardial infarct is another example of a secondary pathology. Other conditions that may well represent illnesses arising at the level of impairment (with possible contributions from levels of disability and handicap) include chronic fatigue syndrome; situational anxiety; post-traumatic stress disorder; and pseudoepilepsy. It is of interest that an intervention at the level of impairment, cognitive behavioural treatment, is effective at reducing the illness experienced in chronic fatigue syndrome[77]; this adds weight to the supposition that this illness has no primary pathological process.

The prediction from the WHO ICIDH model that in some instances illness may arise primarily at the level of impairment is at least plausible. The mechanisms and the relation to changes at the level of pathology are still to be determined. Sometimes the cause may lie within the patients, whereas in other cases external stressors may be responsible. Epidemiological research might help validate this cause of disability and handicap, and also might help to foster rational management of the many patients with these disorders.

132

Conclusions

There is an urgent need for research into the mechanisms of disablement and traditional epidemiological methodology would be an effective approach. The current information is sparse, but does support the hypothesis that the links between pathology, impairment, and disability are weak in individual patients, although there are some important exceptions (spinal cord injury). There may well be cases of patients with disability and impairment but no pathology. There is specifically no information on the relation between combinations of impairments and the resultant disability. There is little information on the importance (or otherwise) of impaired cognition and emotional control in the generation or alleviation of disability. There is little information on how altering the physical, social, and legal environment might affect handicap. A clear understanding of the mechanisms underlying disability might allow a more rational, efficient, and cost effective approach to the management of patients with neurological disability. Research into neurological disability is needed urgently, using traditional epidemiological methods to unravel the extremely complex interrelations.

1 Wood PHN, Badley EM. Contribution of epidemiology to health care planning for people with disabilities. In: Granger CV, Gresham GE, eds. *Functional assessment in rehabilitation medicine.* London: Williams and Wilkins, 1984.

2 Wade DT, Langton-Hewer R. Epidemiology of some neurological diseases with special reference to work load on the NHS. *International Disability Studies* 1986;8:129–37.

3 Wade DT. Designing district disability services—the Oxford experience. *Clinical Rehabilitation* 1990;4:147–58.

4 Wade DT. Stroke (acute cerebrovascular disease). In: Stevens A, Raftery J, eds. *Health care needs assessment. The epidemiologically-based needs assessment reviews.* Oxford: Radcliffe Medical Press, 1994.

5 Wade DT. Policies on the management of patients with head injuries: the experience of the Oxford Region. *Clinical Rehabilitation* 1991;5:141–55.

6 British Society of Rehabilitation Medicine. *A working party report on multiple sclerosis.* London: Royal College of Physicians, 1993.

7 Brown S, Betts T, Chadwick D, Hall B, Shorvon S. An epilepsy needs document. *Seizure* 1993;2:91–103.

8 Leone M, Bottacchi LM, D'Alessandro G, Kustermann S. Hereditary ataxias and paraplegias in Valle d'Aosta, Italy: a study of prevalence and disability. *Acta Neurol Scand* 1995;91:183–7.

9 Perkin GD. An analysis of 7836 successive new out-patient referrals. *J Neurol Neurosurg Psychiatry* 1989;52:447–51.

10 Hopkins A, Menken M, DeFreise G. A record of patient encounters in neurological practice in the United Kingdom. *J Neurol Neurosurg Psychiatry* 1989;52:436–8.

11 Louis ED, Marder K, Cote L, *et al.* Prevalence of a history of shaking in persons 65 years of age and older: diagnostic and functional correlates. *Mov Disord* 1996;**11**:63–9.

12 Knight R, Warren MD. *Physically disabled people living at home: a study of numbers and needs. Report on health and social subjects 13.* London: Department of Health and Social Security; HMSO, 1978.

13 Hanley J, McAndrew L. A survey of the younger chronic sick and disabled in the community in the Lothian region. *International Disability Studies* 1987;**9**:74–7.

14 Martin J, Meltzer H, Elliott D. *The prevalence of disability among adults. Surveys of disability in Great Britain. Report 1.* London: Office of Population Censuses and Surveys; HMSO, 1988.

15 Harrison J. *Severe physical disability. Responses to the challenge of care.* London: Cassell Educational, 1987.

16 Royal College of Physicians. *The young disabled adult.* London: Royal College of Physicians,1986.

17 Prouse P, Ross-Smith K, Brill M, Singh M, Brennan P, Frank A. Community support for young physically handicapped people. *Health Trends* 1991; **23**:105–9.

18 Nagi S. An epidemiology of disability among adults in the USA. *MMFQ/Health and Society* 1976;**439**–67.

19 World Health Organisation. *International classification of impairments, disabilities, and handicaps.* Geneva: WHO, 1980.

20 Duckworth D. The need for a standard terminology and classification of disablement. In: Granger CV, Gresham GE, eds. *Functional assessment in rehabilitation medicine.* London: Williams and Wilkins, 1984.

21 Granger CV. A conceptual model for functional assessment. In: Granger CV, Gresham GE, eds. *Functional assessment in rehabilitation medicine.* London: Williams and Wilkins, 1984.

22 Wade DT. Neurological rehabilitation. In: Kennard C, ed. *Recent advances in clinical neurology.* London: Churchill Livingstone, 1990.

23 Badley EM. An introduction to the concepts and classifications of the international classification of impairments, disabilities and handicaps. *Disabil Rehabil* 1993;**15**:161–78.

24 Wade DT. Measurement in neurological rehabilitation. Oxford: Oxford Medical Publications, 1992.

25 Whyte J. Toward a methodology for rehabilitation research. *Am J Phys Med Rehabil* 1994;**73**:428–35.

26 Bamford J, Sandercock P, Dennis M, Warlow C. Classification and natural history of clinically identifiable subtypes of cerebral infarction. *Lancet* 1991;**337**:1521–6.

27 Allen CMC. *The accurate diagnosis and prognosis of acute stroke. Correlation of clinical features with computed tomographic appearances and functional outcome.* MD thesis, University of Cambridge, 1985.

28 Moller A, Wiedemann G, Rohde U, Backmund H, Sonntag A. Correlates of cognitive impairment and depressive mood disorder in multiple sclerosis. *Acta Psychiatr Scand* 1994;**89**:117–21.

29 Rao SM. Neuropsychology of multiple sclerosis. *Current Opinion in Neurology* 1995;**8**:216–20.

30 Goldberg YP, Telenius H, Hayden MR. The molecular genetics of Huntington's disease. *Current Opinion in Neurology* 1994;**7**:325–32.

31 Morrisey SP, Miller DH, Kendall BE, *et al.* The significance of brain magnetic resonance imaging abnormalities at presentation with clinically isolated syndromes suggestive of multiple sclerosis. *Brain* 1993;**116**:135–46.

134

32 Roberts RC, Shorvon SD, Cox TCS, Gilliat RW. Clinically unsuspected cerebral infarction revealed by computed tomography scanning in late onset epilepsy. *Epilepsia* 1988;**29**:190–4.

33 Kase CS, Wolf PA, Chodosh EH, Zacker HB, Kelly-Hayes M, Kannel WB, *et al*. Prevalence of silent stroke in patients presenting with initial stroke: the Framingham study. *Stroke* 1989;**20**:850–2.

34 Jorgenson HS, Nakayama H, Raaschou HO, Gam J, Olsen TS. Silent infarction in acute stroke patients. Prevalence, localisation, risk factors, and clinical significance: the Copenhagen stroke study. *Stroke* 1994;**25**:97–104.

35 Anderson SW, Damasio H, Jones RD, Tranel D. Wisconsin card sorting test as a measure of frontal lobe damage. *J Clin Exp Neuropsychol* 1991;**13**:909–22.

36 Arnett PA, Rao SM, Bernardin L, Grafman J, Yetkin FZ, Lobeck L. Relationship between frontal lobe lesions and Wisconsin card sorting test performance in patients with multiple sclerosis. *Neurology* 1994;**44**:420–5.

37 Willmes K, Poeck K. To what extent can aphasic syndromes be localised? *Brain* 1993;**116**:1527–40.

38 Rondinelli RD, Murphy JR, Wilson DH, Miller CC. Predictors of functional outcome and resource utilisation in inpatient rehabilitation. *Arch Phys Med Rehabil* 1991;**72**:447–53.

39 Thompson AJ, Kermode AG, MacManus DG, *et al*. Patterns of disease activity in multiple sclerosis: clinical and magnetic resonance imaging study. *BMJ* 1990;**300**:631–4.

40 Khoury SJ, Guttmann CRG, Orav EJ, *et al*. Longitudinal MRI in multiple sclerosis: correlation between disability and lesion burden. *Neurology* 1994;**44**:2120–4.

41 Filippi M, Paty DW, Kappos L, *et al*. Correlations between changes in disability and T2-weighted brain MRI activity in multiple sclerosis: a follow-up study. *Neurology* 1995;**45**:255–60.

42 Miller LS, Miyamoto AT. Computed tomography: its potential as a predictor of functional recovery following stroke. *Arch Phys Med Rehabil* 1979;**60**:108–9.

43 Henon H, Godefroy O, Leys D, Mounier-Vehier F, Lucas C, Rondepierre P, *et al*. Early predictors of death and disability after acute cerebral ischaemic event. *Stroke* 1995;**26**:392–8.

44 Geurts ACH, Mulder TW, Nienhuis B, Rijken RAJ. Dual-task assessment of reorganisation of postural control in persons with lower limb amputation. *Arch Phys Med Rehabil* 1991;**72**:1059–64.

45 Gladman JRF, Harwood DMJ, Barer DH. Predicting the outcome of acute stroke: prospective evaluation of five multivariate models and comparison with simple methods. *J Neurol Neurosurg Psychiatry* 1992;**55**:347–51.

46 Wade DT, Langton-Hewer R. Functional abilities after stroke: measurement, natural history and prognosis. *J Neurol Neurosurg Psychiatry* 1987;**50**:177–82.

47 Bohannon RW. Selected determinants of ambulatory capacity in patients with hemiplegia. *Clinical Rehabilitation* 1989;**3**:47–53.

48 Bendall MJ, Bassey EJ, Pearson MB. Factors affecting walking speed of elderly people. *Age Ageing* 1989;**18**:327–32.

49 Parker VM, Wade DT, Langton-Hewer R. Loss of arm function after stroke: measurement, frequency, and recovery. *International Rehabilitation Medicine* 1986;**8**:69–73.

50 Cockburn J, Smith PT, Wade DT. Influence of cognitive function on social, domestic and leisure activities of community-dwelling older people. *International Disability Studies* 1990;**12**:169–72.

51 Farmer JE, Eakman AM. The relationship between neuropsychological functioning and instrumental activities of daily living following acquired brain injury. *Applied Neuropsychology* 1995;**2**:107–15.

52 Stubgen JP, Lahouter A. Limb girdle muscular dystrophy: weakness and disease duration as predictors of functional impairment. *Muscle Nerve* 1994; **17**:873–80.

53 Cornwall A. The relationship of phonological awareness, rapid naming, and verbal memory to severe reading and spelling disability. *Journal of Learning Disability* 1992;**25**:532–8.

54 Collen FM, Wade DT. Residual mobility problems after stroke. *International Disability Studies* 1991;**13**:12–15.

55 Waters RL, Adkins R, Yakura J, Vigil D. Prediction of ambulatory performance based on motor scores derived from standards of the American Spinal Injury Association. *Arch Phys Med Rehabil* 1994;**75**:756–60.

56 Tatemichi TK, Desmond DW, Mayeux R *et al*. Dementia after stroke: baseline frequency, risks, and clinical features in a hospitalised cohort. *Neurology* 1992;**42**:1185–93.

57 Wade DT, Skilbeck C, Langton-Hewer R. Selected cognitive losses after stroke: frequency, recovery and prognostic importance. *International Disability Studies* 1989;**11**:34–9.

58 Worthington A. Psychological aspects of motor neurone disease: a review. *Clinical Rehabilitation* 1996;**10**:185–94.

59 Brown RG, Marsden CD. How common is dementia in Parkinson's disease? *Lancet* 1984;**2**:1262–5.

60 House A. Depression after stroke. *BMJ* 1987;**294**:76–8.

61 Minden SL, Schiffer RB. Affective disorders in multiple sclerosis. Review and recommendations for clinical research. *Arch Neurol* 1990;**47**:98–104.

62 Lipsey JR, Robinson RG, Pearlson GD, Rao K, Price TR. Nortriptyline treatment of post-stroke depression: a double blind study. *Lancet* 1984;**1**:297–300.

63 Reding MJ, Orto LA, Winter SW, Fortuna IM, Ponte PD, McDowell FH. Anti-depressant therapy after stroke. A double-blind trial. *Arch Neurol* 1986;**43**:763–5.

64 Belcher SA, Clowers MR, Cabanayan AC, Fordyce WE. Activity patterns of married and single people after stroke. *Arch Phys Med Rehabil* 1982;**63**:308–12.

65 Lehmann JF, Condon SM, Price R, deLateur BJ. Gait abnormalities in hemiplegia: their correction by ankle-foot orthoses. *Arch Phys Med Rehabil* 1987;**68**:763–71.

66 Badley EM. The genesis of handicap: definition, models of disablement, and role of external factors. *Disability and Rehabilitation* 1995;**17**:53–62.

67 McDonough PA, Badley EM, Tennant A. Disability, resources, role demands and mobility handicap. *Disability and Rehabilitation* 1995;**17**:159–68.

68 Yardley L, Putman J. Quantitative analysis of factors contributing to handicap and distress in vertiginous patients: a questionnaire study. *Clinical Otolaryngol* 1992;**17**:231–6.

69 Wade DT, Legh-Smith J, Hewer RL. Depressed mood after stroke. A community study of its frequency. *Br J Psychiatry* 1987;**151**:200–5.

70 Ron MA. Somatisation in neurological practice. *J Neurol Neurosurg Psychiatry* 1994;**57**:1161–4.

71 Herbert TB, Cohen S. Depression and immunity: a meta-analytic review. *Psychol Bull* 1993;**113**:472–86.

72 Ader R, Cohen N, Felten D. Psychoneuroimmunology: interactions between the nervous system and the immune system. *Lancet* 1995;**345**:99–103.

73 Phillimore P, Beattie A, Townsend P. Widening inequality of health in northern England, 1981–91. *BMJ* 1994;**308**:1125–8.

74 Smith GD. Income inequality and mortality: why are they related? *BMJ* 1996;**312**:988–9.

75 Diehr P, Diehr G, Koepsell T, Wood R, Beach K, Wolcott B, Tompkins RK. Cluster analysis to determine headache types. *Journal of Chronic Disease* 1982;**35**:623–33.
76 Ziegler DK, Hassanein RS, Couch JR. Headache syndromes suggested by statistical analysis of headache symptoms. *Cephalalgia* 1982;**2**:125–34.
77 Sharpe M, Hawton K, Simkin S, *et al*. Cognitive behaviour therapy for the chronic fatigue syndrome: a randomised controlled trial. *BMJ* 1996;**312**:22–6.

7 The Epilepsies

JOSEMIR SANDER, SIMON SHORVON

> - In developed countries the prevalence of epilepsy is 5-10 per 1000 and the annual incidence 50 per 1000.
> - Age-specific incidence rates appear to be changing. Incidence is decreasing in younger age groups and increasing in older age groups.
> - The incidence of seizure disorders varies geographically.
> - The current syndromic classification of the epilepsies is unsatisfactory for population-based research.

Methodological issues

Diagnostic accuracy and case finding

To carry out epidemiological studies, sensitive and specific diagnostic and case ascertainment methods are essential. In the epilepsies, a problem common to all epidemiological studies is diagnostic accuracy. A number of factors make epilepsy difficult to diagnose with certainty. Epileptic seizures are pleomorphic, although usually stereotyped for a given individual. Unlike most neurological disorders, most patients with seizures do not have permanent physical signs. For most of the time the disorder is "invisible".[1] Thus it can be diagnosed only by taking a history of the index event or by the chance observation of a seizure. The clinical diagnosis is fundamentally a discretionary judgement which may vary depending on the skill and experience of the physician and the quality of witness information available.[2] The EEG is useful in classifying epileptic seizures, but is of only limited help in making the diagnosis.

The differential diagnosis of epilepsy encompasses all causes of transient alterations of consciousness, and in practice both false positive and false negative diagnoses are common. Common sources of confusion are syncope or psychogenic attacks. Syncope is often misdiagnosed as epilepsy at least initially.[1-3] It has also been estimated that as many as 10–20% of chronic cases referred to specialised epilepsy units with seemingly intractable chronic seizures do not have true epileptic attacks.[1 2 4-6] In the case of the non-epileptic attacks, a compounding factor is that some of the patients may also have concomitant epileptic seizures or have had epilepsy in the past. It is now generally accepted that 20–30% of patients developing epilepsy will eventually be classified as sufferers of chronic epilepsy.[7-8] The inclusion of patients with non-epileptic attacks in the latter group may artificially inflate the proportion of chronic cases.[8] By contrast, many patients with epilepsy have the condition for months or years before the correct diagnosis is achieved. In the Rochester study, the time from the first seizure to diagnosis exceeded two years in more than 30% of patients.[9] Similarly, in the UK National General Practice Study of Epilepsy, a population based study of newly diagnosed epilepsy, the diagnosis was unclear six months after entry to the study in 29% of the patients.[10] There has been little acknowledgement of this problem in epidemiological surveys, and diagnostic criteria have been, with a few exceptions, unspecified or loosely defined. A large incidence and prevalence study carried out in Northern Ecuador is one of the few exceptions where clear and reproducible diagnostic definitions were used.[11] Account was taken of diagnostic uncertainties by reporting the findings as a range rather than a single figure. The lower figure of the range was estimated from definite cases identified and the higher figure was derived from all possible cases estimated to exist from diagnostic reviews and quality control procedures.[12]

Even if diagnosis is accurate, case ascertainment poses a variety of problems in the epilepsies. Some patients with epileptic seizures never seek medical attention, either because they ignore or misinterpret the symptoms, or indeed may be unaware of them, and this is particularly true of absence and some minor complex partial seizures.[13] Sometimes the patient or carers may conceal or deny the condition.[13 14] It is likely, therefore, that epidemiological studies of epilepsy, both cross sectional and longitudinal, miss patients unless sensitive screening techniques for all epileptic phenomena are included in the case ascertainment. This has not yet been achieved. It could be argued that patients not presenting to a medical agency should not be considered a problem. This may hold sway in clinical practice but in epidemiology it is important that all cases are included.[15]

The optimum method to obtain accurate incidence, prevalence and outcome data for the epilepsies would be to interview all persons and their close relatives or friends (witnesses) in the proband population to ascertain a history of seizures and to monitor closely the whole population in question for a specified period of time to identify all new cases at the time of onset. All those cases identified would then be followed until death. This approach is, however, unrealistic, and other less satisfactory but feasible methods have to be used.[15]

The most common method of case ascertainment, in the developed world at least, is that of a retrospective review of medical notes. Usually, the case records are reviewed for a mention of seizures, prescription of antiepileptic drugs (AEDs), request for EEG, or a diagnostic index is used.[1] For all the reasons discussed above, there are major sources of inaccuracy, and underreporting is common. The extent of this was clearly shown by a study in Warsaw that found a prevalence rate of 5·1/1000 based on a survey of medical records alone which rose to 10·4/1000 when a sample of 0·5% of the community with their households was added.[13] Similarly, in Guam, incidence rates ranged from 17/100 000 to 35/100 000, and the rates based on field surveys were twice as high as those based on medical records only.[16] In addition, differing diagnostic or therapeutic practices and temporal changes within or between different centres are invariably ignored.[1]

Studies employing record reviews have covered total populations,[17-23] a random sample,[13-24] or selected groups such as sick funds policy holders,[25] army draftees,[26] hospital attenders,[27-28] school children,[29-31] government employees,[32] individuals with learning disabilities,[33] or general practitioners' lists.[34-37] A retrospective case record review may be supplemented by an interview of positively identified cases.[35] A second approach has been the use of a register of cases such as in Rochester, Minnesota[9 38] or Aarhus, Denmark[39] but unless careful precautions are taken, these may suffer exactly the same diagnostic problems as a simple review of existing records. An advantage of a register set up for research purposes is that the methodology may be planned in advance.[1]

An epidemiological approach that does not rely on prior diagnosis is to carry out a community or house to house survey using a screening questionnaire that is sensitive and specific.[40] This strategy works for generalised tonic–clonic seizures and other seizure types with florid clinical symptomatology. For other seizure types, however, this may not be accurate as a pragmatic screening instrument for these seizures has not yet been designed; indeed a recent attempt to design such a questionnaire had to be abandoned due to the low specificity of questions relating to absence seizures and myoclonic seizures that would render any field survey using it impractical.[40]

Community or house to house surveys using a screening questionnaire have been carried out in various locations.[12 13 41-66] Some studies have included the entire population or random samples, and others have selected racial or demographic subgroups or specific age groups. In some investigations, hospital and medical records, public health records, school and institutional records are also surveyed. Of course, such surveys depend crucially on the adequacy of the screening methods (usually administered by non-medically qualified persons), and these are difficult to design. It is important to achieve a balance between sensitivity and specificity, and to date this does not seem to have been satisfactorily achieved.[40] A screening questionnaire and its validation are not easily transferable between different populations due to cultural and social influences and therefore must in all cases be piloted and validated for each population where it will be used. The validation process of a screening instrument has only been reported in full by one study[40] although several other studies have given some information about the process.[13 44 48 50-52 54 55 59 60]

In spite of these possible problems, a screening procedure should, in theory at least, be the optimum method for the detection of all active cases. In practice, inactive cases are likely to be overlooked by all these methods, and a review of primary care records, where these are comprehensive, supplemented by patient examination, is probably the optimum method of identifying inactive patients.[35 36]

Classification

The classifications of epilepsy that are in common usage are unsatisfactory for epidemiological purposes. Commonly cases are categorised according to seizure type and occasionally into broad aetiological categories. As with the diagnosis of epilepsy itself, the classification of seizure type depends primarily on a skilfully obtained seizure description. An internationally agreed classification of seizure types has been proposed, which incorporates EEG data in a way that is inadequately defined and a source of confusion.[67] Even when presented with extensive EEG recordings and clinical data, hospital specialists often fail to agree on seizure type classification,[68] and disagreements concerning seizure classification are frequently voiced.[69][70] Furthermore, the use of EEG in field surveys or retrospective reviews of medical records is often impractical, in which case the international seizure type classification is strictly speaking inapplicable.[71] Many published studies, however, have reported the use of this system, without using EEG data while others have used modified versions of the scheme which do not require EEG data.[11]

As discussed above, epileptic seizures may be a manifestation of many disease entities, and an aetiological classification is of great interest. The relative frequency of different causes may vary in different locations. Cysticercosis is, for instance, the commonest identified cause of epilepsy in Mexico[72-73] and in Ecuador,[74] but is virtually unknown in Europe.

Most studies that have attempted to classify aetiologies have done so in broad aetiological grouping, i.e. symptomatic and cryptogenic or idiopathic. Few cross sectional studies have attempted to classify patients in terms of more strictly defined aetiologies. Reasons for this may be logistical, as in many locations sophisticated investigations are impractical. It is self evident that the successful detection of an aetiological factor depends upon the extent of investigation, and unless this is standardised and specified in any large scale study, evaluation of the results is problematic. The use of the terms "idiopathic epilepsy" and "cryptogenic epilepsy" is a particular source of confusion. "Idiopathic epilepsy" is used by some authors to refer to the primary generalised epilepsies which have a genetic component with strictly defined clinical and EEG findings,[75] but by others to refer to any case in which aetiology has not been established. This may make comparisons impossible, as the majority of the cryptogenic epilepsies differ in many respects from primary generalised epilepsy.

An International Classification of Epilepsies, Epileptic syndromes and related disorders has been proposed by the International League Against Epilepsy (ILAE).[76] This scheme, which is perhaps appropriate for use in tertiary referral centres, is cumbersome and difficult to apply in a field study or in retrospective surveys. Probably as a result of this it has seldom been used in any large population study.[77] The Commission of Epidemiology and prognosis of the ILAE in their recent guidelines for epidemiological studies on epilepsy offers a simplified version of the scheme and its use should be encouraged.[78] These guidelines define idiopathic epilepsies as being partial or generalised epileptic syndromes with particular clinical and EEG characteristics and a genetic component. The term "cryptogenic epilepsies" should be reserved for unprovoked partial or generalised seizures in which no factor associated with an increased risk of seizures has been identified and the term "symptomatic" for seizures associated with a known risk factor.[78]

Further difficulties arise concerning the definition of "epilepsy". The inclusion of single seizures, neonatal seizures, febrile seizures, acute symptomatic seizures and inactive seizures may vary from study to study, and this may alter any rate by two or three fold. The Commission guidelines lay down clear definitions for all relevant variables, and rigorous adherence to these in future epidemiological work will address some of these problems. It defines epilepsy, epileptic seizures, single seizures, active and inactive epilepsy, febrile convulsions, status epilepticus, and nonepileptic events. It also defines aetiological categories and recommends that the extent of investigations carried out in any study be fully disclosed.

Another source of difficulty in prevalence studies is the patient with inactive epilepsy. It is now clear that in most people with epilepsy the seizures cease[8 35 79] but there is no general agreement as to what length of remission should occur before a patient is no longer designated as an active case. Some influential investigators have taken the view that "once an epileptic always an epileptic";[80] others have defined epilepsy as a condition in which a seizure has occurred in the preceding year, two, three, or five years. Some investigators have taken treatment status into account, with patients in remission included if they are still taking AEDs. Most reports, however, appear not to have considered this problem, and indeed it is often difficult to determine if reported rates, particularly of prevalence, are for the active condition or lifetime rates. In recognition of this problem the Commission's guidelines have also defined epileptic syndromes in terms of activity.[78] An active case is defined as a person with epilepsy who has had at least one epileptic seizure in the previous five years regardless of treatment. Inactive cases are defined as remission with treatment (a person with epilepsy with no seizures for more than five years and receiving treatment at the time of ascertainment) or remission without treatment (a person with epilepsy with no seizures for more than five years and not receiving treatment at the time of ascertainment).

Geographic distribution

Incidence

Most of the incidence studies were retrospective and were carried out in the developed world. To date no prospective general population based study of the incidence of epileptic syndromes has been reported. There have, however, been a few clinic based studies of the incidence rates of specific syndromes, for instance photosensitive epilepsy.[81]

Case ascertainment has usually been carried out from medical records or from hospital clinics, as for instance in the studies from Nigata City, Japan,[82] Iceland,[17] Guam,[16] Warsaw,[13] Copparo, Italy,[21] but some have covered the whole population of an area as in Umea, Sweden.[83] In some investigations, these were augmented by a medical re-examination.[13 17 84] In the Guam studies[16] and in the Warsaw studies,[13] a representative household sample was also included. The studies from Rochester, Minnesota, and Aarhus, Denmark, have used a retrospective research register.[9 38 39] In five studies from the developing world a community based house to house survey was used and incidence rates derived from cases whose seizures started in the year prior to the survey. Two of these studies took place in Ecuador[12 55] and the others in China,[58] Chile,[63] and Tanzania.[64] Studies from groups of general practitioners have been carried out in the United Kingdom,[34 37 85] and they have used the number of patients registered in each practice as denominators instead of the more commonly used census figures. A particular problem in these investigations was the wide variation from practice to practice, suggesting that some general practitioners may have been more assiduous in their registration than others.

The annual incidence rates reported vary between 11/100 000 in Norway[18] and 230/100 000 in Ecuador[55], although most lie between 40 and 70/100 000 (table 7.1). The highest figures are from populations in developing countries,[12 55 63] and this has been a consistent finding: almost all studies coming from such countries have reported incidence rates of over 100/100 000 while those

Table 7.1:   Published incidence and prevalence rates of
epilepsy in the general population in different countries

Country	Incidence (per 100 000)	Prevalence (per 1000)
Brazil[97]	n/a	13*
Colombia[46]	n/a	19.5*
Chile[63]	113	11.5–17.7
China[58]	35	4.4
Ecuador[12 51 55]	122–190	6.7–8.0[12]
	n/a	7.1–17.0[54]
	230	9.3[55]
Ethiopia[62]	n/a	5.2
Faroes[96]	42	7.6
Guatemala[66]	n/a	5.8
Iceland[17]	26	5.2
Italy[21]	33	6.2
India[60 98]	n/a	3.6[60]
	n/a	2.5[98]
Libya[28]	n/a	2.3
Nigeria[51]	n/a	5.3
Norway[20]	33	3.5
Pakistan[65]	n/a	7.4–14.8
United Kingdom[85 35 36]	63	4.2[85]
	52	5.3[35]
	48	4.3[36]
United States[9 95]	n/a	6.8[95]
	54	5.7[9]
Tanzania[64]	73–140	5.1–37.0

*lifetime prevalence

from the developed world are usually between 40 and 70/100 000.
In the developed world the classic studies of incidence are those
from Rochester, Minnesota, that are based on the Mayo Clinic
Linkage system[9 38] and that have assessed incidence from 1935 to
1984. Age adjusted annual incidence rates have hovered between
40 and 50/100 000, and few changes were seen in overall rates
although it was observed that over time the incidence decreased in
children and increased in the elderly. In the developing world a
study from semi-rural Ecuador, where meticulous care was taken
with methodological issues, reported an annual incidence rate
between 122 and 190/100 000.[12]

Prevalence rates

As cross sectional data are more easily obtained there are many
more studies of the prevalence of epileptic seizures than of
incidence; indeed, studies have been carried out in more than 25
countries in all five continents.[9 13 16–21 31–32 34–36 42–52 54–57 60 63–66 82 86–102] Most
studies giving data on incidence also report prevalence, and there
are additional investigations, some of which have been restricted
to selected populations such as army draftees,[26] sick fund policy

145

holders,[25] mine workers,[103] school children[48 90 104] the elderly,[105] or birth cohorts of children.[84 106]

As is the case with incidence rates, reported prevalence rates are also very variable, and rates as high as 57/1000 and as low as 1·5/1000 have been given for active epilepsy (table 7.1). The average lifetime prevalence rates reported in these studies is 18·5/1000 (range 2.8–44/1000) for children only and 10·3/1000 (range: 1·5–57/1000) for all ages. The problems of case ascertainment have been largely ignored in a number of these studies, and no doubt this is partially responsible for the 30 fold range in prevalence rates. The importance of definition can be illustrated by the study of 6000 patients from one general practice in southern England, where a lifetime prevalence of 20·3/1000 was found for all cases (including single, recurrent, active and inactive cases but excluding febrile seizures) and 17·0 for those with recurrent seizures only, 10·5 for those with active epilepsy (defined as a seizure in the previous two years) and/or on treatment and 5·3/1000 for those with active epilepsy only.[35]

In relatively unselected populations, most studies in both the developing and the developed world have found the point prevalence of active epilepsy to lie between 4 and 10/1000.[9 12 13 17 21 22 24 31 35–36 51 60 62 65 66 85 95–96] For prevalence studies, case finding methods may be usefully combined and the population investigated at both community and hospital levels by screening questionnaire and medical examination. Many investigations may have underestimated the prevalence of epilepsy, and even if single seizures, febrile convulsions, seizures with acute illnesses, neonatal seizures and inactive epilepsy are excluded, rates for chronic epilepsy of around 5–10/1000 are probably applicable to all general populations in both the developed and the developing world.

There have been a number of studies originating in developing countries which reported high prevalence rates for epilepsy. These were from Tanzania,[87 107] Nigeria,[50] Liberia,[93] Chile,[63] Brazil,[108] and Panama.[109] Indeed, the latter study reported the highest recorded prevalence rate of 57/1000; this was a study of 337 tribesmen with a concomitant high incidence of febrile convulsion. One problem with these, however, is that they were mostly small scale studies of selected or isolated populations which may have high rates of genetic or rare degenerative diseases or a high prevalence of parasitic diseases.[8]

Most large scale studies of populations in the developing world have reported overall prevalence rates for active epilepsy around or below 10/1000;[12 51 58 60 62 65 66] some of these studies have, however, reported differential rates for urban and rural areas, usually with higher rates in the latter.[12 65] This is clearly illustrated in a study from southern Pakistan, where a prevalence rate for active epilepsy of 9·9/1000 for the area as a whole was reported; in the rural areas this was, however, 15/1000 in contrast to 7·4/1000 in the urban population surveyed.[65] Similarly, in Ecuador a minimum lifetime prevalence of 14·3/1000 was reported for an Andean region; corresponding values for the urban and rural areas were respectively 9/1000 and 15·4/1000.[12] Furthermore, in this study the area surveyed was divided in two distinct subregions: an upper region situated at an average of 2500–3200 m above sea-level inhabited primarily by people of Amerindian background, and the other a temperate region situated at 1500–2000 m above sea level and with a population of African extraction. The lifetime prevalence of epilepsy was much lower in the higher area than in the lower region: 11·2/1000 against 24·8/1000. Other studies have also reported differing prevalence rates from within study areas. In Tanzania, an overall prevalence rate of 10/1000 was reported for a rural district consisting of 11 villages; rates varied among the various villages and a prevalence range of five to 37/1000 was found.[64] The difference reported in these studies from Pakistan, Ecuador and Tanzania seem unlikely to be artefactual or attributable to differential case ascertainment between the region as each study used identical methods, study design and diagnostic confirmation in each area. No clear aetiological reason for these geographic variations in the prevalence in contiguous geographic areas was identified. These differences are of great potential importance, for herein may lie a clue to aetiology, and they may indeed possibly provide the basis for the prevention of epilepsy in rural areas. Future epidemiological work should be carried out to identify the reasons for these marked differences, including studies of the prevalence and case control studies of neurocysticercosis and other parasitic diseases in rural areas of developing countries.

Lifetime prevalence

Cumulative incidence or lifetime prevalence rates are much higher than the incidence or the prevalence of active epilepsy, and on the basis of available figures it is generally agreed that 1.5–5% of any population will have non-febrile seizures at some time.[8 9 12 17 35 36 38 39 83 85 108] This finding applies to patients both in the developed and in the developing world, where the incidence seem to be higher and where AED treatment is not usually available. From the difference between lifetime prevalence and the point prevalence of active epilepsy it is obvious that most patients developing epilepsy will cease to have seizures or die. It is likely that in most patients with seizure disorders the condition remits, however, it is known that the epilepsies are associated with an increased mortality particularly, but not exclusively, with symptomatic cases.[110-113] Patients with chronic epilepsy seem to be particularly at risk, but the impact of mortality in the prevalence of epilepsy, and the extent to which the difference in lifetime and point prevalence rates is due to mortality, have not yet been fully appraised.[114-115]

In the developed world the overall good prognosis for seizure control is now attributed mainly to the widespread and early use of AEDs.[8 112] The suggestion has been made, however, that a significant number of patients developing an epileptic syndrome will enter a permanent remission regardless of AED treatment.[8] Support for this proposition has come from analysis of epidemiological data arising from the developing world where, despite the lack of AEDs, a significant number of patients enter long term remission.[116] In addition, it is well recognised that a number of epileptic syndromes, for instance benign rolandic epilepsy and benign familial neonatal convulsions, have an excellent outcome independent of AED treatment.[112] This is an area that requires further work, as, if this lack of effect of AEDs on prognosis is true on a wider basis, a change in the routine management of epilepsy may be necessary. If patients with an inherently good prognosis for their epileptic syndrome could be identified at the onset of their condition, the option of no treatment or only very short courses of treatment (to avoid seizure related accidents and morbidity) could become clear alternatives. If by the same token, inherently bad prognosis syndromes could be identified earlier, more aggressive management may limit the 'progression' of the disorder.

Demographic and secular trends

Little attention has been directed to changes in epidemiological rates over time. In most studies, age specific incidence rates are bimodally distributed with the highest peak in the first decade and within this decade in the first year of life. The rates fall in the second decade and remain low in early and mid adult life only to increase in late life when the second peak is observed. This, however, might be changing as some interesting shifts have been seen lately.[117] In southeast England the incidence of epilepsy in children declined from 152/100 000 in the period of 1974 to 1983 to 61/100 000 in the years from 1984–93 while increasing in the elderly over the same period.[36] Similarly, in Rochester, Minnesota, the incidence of seizure disorders has decreased in children over time while it increased in the elderly to a point that the highest peak in now seen in people over the age of 75 years.[38] In Sweden it has recently been reported that the highest incidence of epileptic seizures is now in people over 65 years of age: 139/100 000 while the overall incidence rate for epilepsy is 56/100 000.[83] The UK National General Practice Study of Epilepsy, a study of incident cases of epilepsy, found that only a quarter of all cases recruited were under 15 years old when one would expect over 40% of new cases in this age bracket if previous age specific incidence data are correct. In this study over a quarter of the patients identified were 60 years old or older.[10 118] In addition, one study has also recently reported changes in the prevalence of epilepsy in the same population over time: the prevalence of active epilepsy declined from 5·3/1000 in 1983 to 4·3/1000 10 years later.[36] No clear explanation for these changes has yet been advanced. In children speculation has centred on the role of improved prenatal care and the adoption of healthier lifestyles by expectant mothers, leading to a decrease in neuronal migration defects and to a reduction in the incidence of birth hypoxia.[112] In the elderly it is presumed that an increase in life expectancy allied to cerebrovascular diseases is responsible for the increase observed. This seems paradoxical, however, as the incidence of cerebrovascular diseases has decreased in the community over the last two decades.[38]

Clinical characteristics

Many studies have found the majority of patients to have generalised seizures, and proportions as high as 88% have been reported.[58] This is, however, likely to be due to such methodological problems as described above. Studies where particular care was taken with seizure classification and EEG was

149

used, the majority of patients had partial seizures with or without secondary generalization and this is also the experience of most tertiary referral centres. In Rochester, Minnesota, 66% of the patients had partial seizures,[9] and in the Warsaw field study 65% of patients were reported to have had partial seizures.[13] In the large population-based Ecuadorian study, seizures were classified without the use of EEG, and half of patients were reported to have had partial seizures.[12 13] In the UK National General Practice study of epilepsy where routine investigations were applied, 52% of patients had partial seizures, 39% generalised seizures, and the remaining were unclassifiable.[10]

In the majority of studies, only two seizure types are at all common: tonic-clonic convulsions, and partial seizures with or without secondary generalisation. Other seizure types, i.e. generalised absence, tonic and atonic seizures, and myoclonic seizures are uncommon. Generalised absence, for instance is usually reported in less than 2% of patients.[15] Although this is a seizure type known to all medical students and practitioners, it is rare in population terms. The patient presenting with an absence is much more likely to have partial seizures than true generalised absence attacks, although these are often confused. In addition, for the diagnosis of true generalised absence seizures, an EEG recording showing three per second spike and waves discharges is necessary. Some studies that have reported the presence of generalised absences did not include EEG as part of the methodology.[15]

The present scheme for seizure classification is unsatisfactory and not suitable for field studies where the use of EEG is impractical. The categorisation of seizure type is often difficult, and there seems to be little doubt that partial seizures are often underreported. Many so called generalised seizures are in fact secondarily generalised and should be categorised as partial, and the detection of a partial onset may depend on the skill of the investigator or the extent of investigation. The studies showing the highest proportion of partial seizures are those in which medical services are the most sophisticated. Thus, although this classification has often been said to have been used in large scale surveys, the reported seizure classification should be viewed with caution. Another point to note is the almost complete absence of unclassified convulsions in published reports which purport to have used the international classification. In hospital practice about one third of cases are unclassifiable.[1]

Only a few population-based studies have reported on seizure frequency and severity. Indeed, very often it is difficult to ascertain, from study reports, how many cases have qualified as cases only due to the usage of AEDs. In one large study of prevalent cases in use of AED in a developed country where this information was provided, 46% of patients were reported to have been seizure free in the previous year, 33% had between one and 12 seizures a year and the remaining more than one seizure a month, 8% of whom had more than 50 seizures a year.[119] In a prevalent population in a developing country, where AED treatment was not generally available and only 15% of patients were using drugs at the time of the survey, 45% of patients were reported to have had less than 10 seizures prior to the survey, 14% between 10 and 100 seizures, and the remaining 26% more than 100 seizures.[116]

The frequency of epilepsy in a population of 100 000 in a developed country based on the figures discussed above is given in table 7.2.

Risk factors, aetiologies and the heterogeneity of the epilepsies

Risk factors and aetiology

From hospital and clinic studies it is well known that the range of aetiologies in the epilepsies varies in different age groups and also according to geographic location. Congenital, developmental and genetic conditions are associated with epilepsy in childhood, adolescence and in young adults. In the elderly, cerebrovascular disease is common. Head trauma, sporadic CNS infection and tumours may occur at any age, although the latter is more likely to occur over the age of 40. In certain areas endemic infections that are associated with epileptic seizures are common. The aetiology

Table 7.2: *The frequency of epilepsy in a population of 100 000 in a developed country*

New cases of epilepsy each year (incidence)	40–70
Cases of active epilepsy (prevalence)	500–1000
Cases who ever had epilepsy	2100–5000
Seizure frequency for those with active epilepsy	
No seizures for more than 12 month:	230–4 60
Between 1 and 12 seizures/year	165–330
Between 12–50 seizures/year	65–130
More than 50 seizures/year	40–80

of epilepsy may be multifactorial, and it has been suggested that an acquired condition maybe more likely to occur if an inherited predisposition is present.[2] The relative contribution of each of these potential causes for the aetiology of the epilepsies in the general population has, however, not yet been formally ascertained.

In most field investigations, a putative aetiology for the epilepsy was found in only about 1/4 or 1/3 of cases. In the Rochester, Minnesota study,[9] 5% were due to head trauma, 5% to cerebrovascular diseases, 4% to brain tumour, 4% to congenital or genetic abnormalities, and 3% to infectious diseases, while in the study from Copparo (which has one of the highest percentages of cases with known aetiology) 20% were said to be secondary to perinatal injuries, 7% to head trauma, 5% to infective diseases, 4% to cerebrovascular diseases, 2% to brain tumour, and in 61% no cause was found.[21] In Ecuador, no putative cause for the seizures was identified in at least 73% of the patients.[12] Likely aetiologies were estimated in the remaining 27% of patients, and these included birth trauma (9%), head injury (7%), neurocysticercosis (3%), and cerebrovascular diseases (3%). In the UK NGPSE, seizures were classified as idiopathic or cryptogenic in 72%, remote symptomatic in 25%, and the remaining 3% were associated with neurological deficits present at birth.[10] The commonest putative aetiology in this study was cerebrovascular disease. Overall 16% of all patients had this as the cause of their epilepsy but this rose to 49% in the age group over 60 years. A similar finding has been reported from Sweden: cerebrovascular diseases were responsible for 30% of all cases of epilepsy in adults, but this increased to 46% in those aged 60 or over.[83]

It is self evident that the more extensive the investigation, the more likely aetiological factors are to be identified. To what extent this would modify the findings of a large scale epidemiological investigation is uncertain. MRI identifies a very much higher rate of positive causes in hospital based surveys, but in field surveys or in retrospective record reviews it is, of course, inapplicable.[120] Indeed, no population based study of epilepsy with modern neuroimaging as part of the study design has yet been reported. Because of this, the true incidence of symptomatic epilepsies in general populations is unknown and is likely to be much higher than that found in the epidemiological studies cited above. No epidemiologically based study yet accurately describes the range of aetiologies of epilepsy. This deficiency urgently needs to be corrected and is a vital prerequisite to sensitive case control investigations of relative risk.

Sex

Most reports show slightly higher rates in males than in females.[1] The suggestion that this is due to a higher incidence of head trauma has never been formally confirmed, and the low overall incidence of posttraumatic epilepsy makes this unlikely.[121 122] Syncope and psychogenic attacks are much more common in females than in males, and the potential for misdiagnosis in epilepsy in females is greater.[4] Consultation rates from general practices in the United Kingdom, for instance, show that women consult their general practitioner for episodes of disturbed consciousness of any sort twice as often as males.[123]

Race and socio-economic status

There are several small scale reports showing high rates in black African populations.[50 86 87 93] In Ecuador, the prevalence of seizures was much higher in a population predominantly of African descent than in a neighbouring population made up mostly of Amerindians.[12] A higher prevalence rate for Afro-Americans than for whites was reported in two studies of American school children.[27 124] A similar finding was reported in adults from a census of neurological diseases in a biracial population of Copiah County in the south of the United States.[95] Similarly, US mortality data suggest that the prevalence of epilepsy in non-whites is twice that of whites in America.[125] A lower standard of perinatal care might be relevant, and the infant mortality rates among black people in America are twice that of white people.[27 126] Indeed, data from other developed countries and also from developing countries suggest higher prevalence rates in the lower socioeconomic classes,[17 34 46 63 127] but no hard evidence for this suggestion has yet been unveiled. Case control studies to address this issue are also needed.

The heterogeneity of the epilepsies

A fundamental issue, often glossed over in the epidemiological literature, is that of the heterogeneity of the epilepsies.[8] Many

153

different conditions, with differing causes and outcomes may express themselves solely by the occurrence of recurrent epileptic seizures. Epilepsy is a collection of syndromes and conditions rather than a single disease, but most studies have reported on 'epilepsy' as a whole or according to seizure type rather than by any more meaningful classification. An analogy can be drawn with anaemia.[128] If the epidemiology of anaemia was studied as if it were a single disorder, it is unlikely that useful aetiological data would ever arise.

The syndromes of idiopathic epilepsy

Even the "idiopathic" epilepsies, which are often considered homogeneous, include conditions with differing incidence and outcome.[112] Thus, generalised absence epilepsy, epilepsy with generalised tonic-clonic convulsions on awakening, and juvenile myoclonic epilepsy are all well recognised syndromes under the rubric of the generalised idiopathic epilepsies. These conditions probably have different genetic mechanisms and may have different natural histories. A 24-fold difference in the cumulative incidence of generalised absence epilepsy has been reported between populations in Sweden and Japan, perhaps due to genetic differences.[15] These aetiologically important factors would be obscured by epidemiological studies that categorised them all under idiopathic epilepsy.

It is self evident but often overlooked, that classification by seizure type alone is not sufficient to allow a classification by syndrome. Generalised tonic-clonic seizures (GTC) are characteristic of many epileptic syndromes. GTC can occur in acute symptomatic epilepsy, generalised epilepsy, whether idiopathic or symptomatic, and in all forms of localisation-related epilepsy. The clinical characteristics of partial seizures also reveal little of aetiological or prognostic value. Seizures represent an expression of an underlying pathology the cause of which is not revealed in the phenomenology of the symptom. Epidemiological studies have, however, typically relied heavily on seizure characteristics as the key epilepsy variable.

Many epilepsy syndromes can only be diagnosed with the benefit of several years of follow-up. Cross-sectional studies will inevitably misclassify a significant number of cases. Studies done before access to modern investigation techniques do not reflect current thinking about the aetiology of epilepsy. The same also applies to field studies, particularly in developing countries, in which even EEG is often not practical.

The need for case control studies to investigate aetiology

Studies have suggested that there are geographic differences in the incidence of epilepsy, with a higher incidence in the developing world. It is often implied that infections of the CNS are partly responsible for this increased incidence and this might well be true as many CNS infective agents are associated with both acute symptomatic seizures and seizures in the aftermath of infection.[129][130] Frequently, studies from the developing world link a high prevalence of some local infectious disease with epilepsy but most of these studies lack sufficient controls to confirm conclusively that the infections are the underlying cause. In Ecuador, Peru, Brazil and Mexico, for instance, neurocysticercosis is prevalent in a large number of attenders of neurological clinics, many of whom may have epilepsy.[73][74][129-134] Post mortem and other studies suggest that asymptomatic cysticercosis is also relatively common.[129][135] What is unknown, however, is the prevalence of epilepsy in all people who harbour cysticerci in their brain. No adequate large scale study of neurocysticercosis, on a population basis, has ever been carried out to ascertain attributable risk. Other parasitic disorders such as malaria,[129][130][136][137] schistosomiasis,[138] paragonimiasis,[129][130][136] or American trypanosomiasis[63][129][139] have also been implicated as risk factors for subsequent epilepsy, but again this has not yet been substantiated. Another possible explanation for the finding of high prevalence rates in geographically isolated clusters would be genetically determined syndromes,[8] but this also lacks confirmation.

Another important area of uncertainty is the role of neuronal migration disorders and other developmental abnormalities of the cerebral cortex in the aetiology of the epilepsies in the general population in both developed and developing countries. These are now well established as associated with chronic epilepsy in hospital attenders.[140][141] It is, however, not known what the prevalence of these conditions is in the population at large to enable an estimation of relative risk. By the same token, the finding of hippocampal sclerosis in patients with chronic partial epilepsy is associated with a history of febrile convulsion between age 3 months and 5 years in over two thirds of the cases.[142] Epilepsy, however, develops in less than 3% of children who experience a

155

febrile convulsion with no prior neurological abnormalities, and the risk factors for this are known.[124 142] It is still not known how common hippocampal sclerosis is in the general population or even among those who as youngsters experienced febrile convulsions but did not subsequently develop chronic epilepsy.

Syndromic classification

Two difficulties can be foreseen with a "syndromic approach" to the neuroepidemiology of the epilepsies. Firstly, the present syndromic classification is provisional. Recent advances in neuroimaging and neurogenetics are likely to identify further syndromes. For example, Familial Autosomal Dominant Frontal Lobe Epilepsy recently became characterised clinically and shortly thereafter was linked to a specific genetic cause in some families.[143] Other new disorders include the milder forms of neuronal migration disorders associated with epilepsy.[140 141] Secondly, there are a number of questions that epidemiology in its present form can not answer, for example, the reason why, in pathologically defined conditions, the response to treatment and final outcome is not always the same. This seems to indicate that factors other than gross pathology influence outcome. Cavernous angiomas, for instance, cause epilepsy in less than 70% of patients identified.[144] Why do some individuals with lesions in similar locations develop epilepsy and others not? Furthermore, some who develop seizures respond to drug treatment, whereas others develop intractable epilepsy. The risk of epilepsy after severe non-penetrating head injury is about 20% at five years; some patients or sufferers respond to drug treatment while others develop intractable epilepsy.[121] There is anecdotal evidence that some people with epilepsy of temporal lobe type associated with hippocampal sclerosis respond favourably to certain AEDs, whilst others fail to respond to any drug. Thus, presently "aetiologies" are not the sole determinant of outcome and response to treatment as other unknown factors must exist. Current epidemiological studies are likely to fail to define completely the epileptic substrate. Further research at a neurobiological level is required before progress can be made. Any future research to have an impact must also take into account the advances in neurogenetics and neuroimaging that so far have not been used to any significant extent in epidemiological work in the epilepsies.

Conclusions

Little is known about the true epidemiology of the different epileptic syndromes in the general population, as definitive studies are lacking. However, data based on seizure types suggest that the epilepsies are common, with an incidence between 40 and 200/100 000 depending on geographic location. Despite this high incidence the overall prevalence lies between 0·5% and 1% in the general population. It may be more common in specific age groups, i.e. children and elderly people, in particular geographic locations for genetic or environmental reasons. Changes in the age specific incidence may be occurring with a shift to the older age groups. Individuals who develop epilepsy not complicated by an underlying neurological disorder have a good prognosis for full seizure control, although the full impact of mortality on the outcome of the epilepsies in the general population has not yet been fully assessed.

To extend our knowledge in this area future studies need to be large scale, general population based prospective incidence studies of the different epileptic syndromes with comprehensive case ascertainment, accurate diagnosis and sound aetiological assignment. Cohorts of patients so identified should then be prospectively followed to determine accurately overall prognosis for seizure control and mortality, in tandem with analytic case control studies to quantify aetiological risk factors. Further cross sectional studies are unlikely to be helpful. Specific questions that require investigation include: the quantification of possible geographic differences in the incidence and the relative contribution of various aetiologies to the difference, the cause of possible changes in the age-specific incidence, and accurate syndrome specific incidence rates. In addition, further studies to delineate the spectrum of epileptic syndromes should be strongly encouraged.

The authors are grateful to Drs M F O'Donoghue, O C Cockerell, N Bharucha and J Duncan for discussions and comments on the concepts discussed in this review.

1 Sander JWAS, Shorvon SD. Incidence and prevalence studies in epilepsy and their methodological problems: a review. *J Neurol Neurosurg Psychiat* 1987;50:829–39.
2 Nashef L. Definitions, aetiologies and diagnosis. In: Shorvon SD, Dreifuss F, Fish D, Thomas D. eds. *The treatment of epilepsy*. Oxford: Blackwell 1996:66–96.

3 Lempert T. Recognising syncope: pitfalls and surprises. *J R Soc Med* 1996;**89**:372–5.

4 Duncan JS. Diagnosis—is it epilepsy? In: Duncan JS, Shorvon SD, Fish DR. eds. *Clinical Epilepsy*. Edinburgh: Churchill Livingstone 1995:1–24.

5 Trimble MR, Ring HA. Psychological and psychiatric aspects of epilepsy. In: Duncan JS, Shorvon SD, Fish DR. eds. *Clinical Epilepsy*. Edinburgh: Churchill Livingstone 1995:321–48.

6 Lesser R. Psychogenic seizures. *Neurology* 1996;**46**:1499–507.

7 Shorvon SD. Chronic epilepsy. *BMJ* 1991;**302**:363–6.

8 Sander JWAS. Some aspect of the prognosis of the epilepsies. *Epilepsia* 1993;**34**:1007–16.

9 Hauser WA, Kurland LT. The epidemiology of epilepsy in Rochester, Minnesota, 1935 through 1967. *Epilepsia* 1975;**16**:1–66.

10 Sander JWAS, Hart YM, Johnson AL, Shorvon SD. The National General Practice Study of Epilepsy: Newly diagnosed seizures in a general population. *Lancet* 1990;**336**:1267–71.

11 Placencia M, Suarez J, Crespo F, Shorvon SD, Sander JWAS *et al*. A large scale study of epilepsy in Ecuador: methodological aspects. *Neuroepidemiology* 1992;**11**:71–84.

12 Placencia M, Shorvon SD, Paredes V, Bimos C, Sander JWAS, Cascante SM. Epileptic seizures in an Andean region of Ecuador: incidence and prevalence and regional variation. *Brain* 1992;**115**:771–82.

13 Zielinski JJ. *Epidemiology and Medico-Social Problems of Epilepsy in Warsaw (Poland)*. Final report on research program no. 19-P-58325-F-01. Warsaw: Psychoneurological Institute 1974.

14 Beran RG, Michelazzi J, Hall L, Tsimnadis P, Loh S. False-Negative response rate in epidemiological studies to define prevalence ratios of epilepsy. *Neuroepidemiology* 1985;**4**:82–5.

15 Sander JWAS. The epidemiology and prognosis of typical absence seizures. In: Duncan JS, Panayiotopoulos CP. eds. *The typical absences and related epileptic syndromes*. Edinburgh: Churchill Livingstone 1994:135–41.

16 Stanhope JM, Brody JA, Brink E. Convulsions among the Chamorro people of Guam, Mariana Island. *Am J Epidem* 1972;**95**:292–8.

17 Gudmundsson G. Epilepsy in Iceland. *Acta Neurol Scand* 1966;**43**:S–25.

18 Krohn W. A study of epilepsy in northern Norway, its frequency and character. *Acta Psychiat Scand* 1961;**36**:S215–25.

19 Leibowitz U, Alter M. Epilepsy in Jerusalem, Israel. *Epilepsia* 1968;**9**:87–105.

20 de Graaf AS. Epidemiological aspects of epilepsia in northern Norway. *Epilepsia* 1974;**15**:291–9.

21 Granieri E, Rosati G, Tola R, *et al*. A descriptive study of epilepsy in the district of Copparo, Italy 1964–78. *Epilepsia* 1983;**24**:502–14.

22 Keranen T, Riekkinen PJ, Sillanpaa M. Incidence and prevalence of epilepsy in adults in Eastern Finland. *Epilepsia* 1989;**30**:413–21.

23 Maremmani C, Rossi G, Bonucelli U, Murri L. Descriptive epidemiological study of epileptic syndromes in a district of north-west Tuscany, Italy. *Epilepsia* 1991;**32**:294–98.

24 Brewis M, Poskanzer D, Rolland C, *et al*. Neurological diseases in a English city. *Acta Neurologica Scandinavica* 1966;43(S–24):1–89.

25 Wajsbort J, Haral N. Alfandary I. A study of the epidemiology of chronic epilepsy in Northern Israel. *Epilepsia* 1967;**8**:105–16.

26 Jallon P. Evaluation du taux de prevalence de l'epilepsie dans un centre de selection de l'armee. *Rev Neurol Paris* 1991;**147**:319–22.

27 Shamansky S, Glaser G. Socio-economic characteristics of childhood seizure disorders in the New Haven area: an epidemiological study. *Epilepsia* 1979;**20**:457–74.

28 Sridharan R, Radhakrishnan K, Ashok PP, Mousa ME. Epidemiological and clinical study of epilepsy in Benghazi, Libya. *Epilepsia* 1986;**27**:60–65.

29 Cooper JE. Epilepsy in a longitudinal survey of 5,000 children. *BMJ* 1965;**1**:1020–2.

30 Costeff H, Convulsions in childhood: their natural history and indications for treatment. *N Engl J Med* 1965;**273**:1410–13.

31 Cavazzuti GB. Epidemiology of different types of epilepsy in school age children of Modena, Italy. *Epilepsia* 1980;**21**:57–62.

32 Olivares L. Epilepsy in Mexico: a population study. In: Milton A. Hauser WA. eds. *The Epidemiology of Epilepsy: a workshop*. NINDS Monograph no. 14. Washington: DHEW. 1972.

33 Forsgren L, Edvinsson S, Blomquist HK, Heijbel J, Sidenvall R. Epilepsy in a population of mentally retarded children and adults. *Epilepsy Res* 1990;**6**:234–48.

34. Pond D, Bidwell B, Stein L. A survey of 14 general practices: Psychiatria, Neurologia, *Neurochirurgia* 1960;**63**:217–36

35 Goodridge DMG, Shorvon SD. Epilepsy in a population of 6000. *BMJ* 1983;**287**:641–7.

36 Cockerell OC, Eckle I, Goodridge DMG, Sander JWAS, Shorvon SD. Epilepsy in a population of 6,000 re-examined: secular trends in first attendance rates, prevalence and prognosis. *J Neurol Neurosurg Psychiat* 1995;**58**:570–6.

37 Cockerell OC, Sander JWAS, Brodie D, Goodridge DGM, Shorvon SD. Neurological conditions in a defined population: the results of a pilot study in two general practices. *Neuroepidemiology* 1996;**15**:73–82.

38 Hauser AW, Annegers JF, Kurland LT. Incidence of epilepsy and unprovoked seizures in Rochester, Minnesota 1935–1984. *Epilepsia* 1993;**34**:453–68.

39 Juul-Jensen P, Foldspang A. Natural history of epileptic seizures. *Epilepsia* 1983;**24**:391–4.

40 Placencia M, Sander JWAS, Shorvon SD, Ellison RH, Suarez S, Cascante SM. Validation of a screening questionnaire for the detection of epileptic seizures in epidemiological studies. *Brain* 1992;**115**:783–94.

41 Lessell S, Torres JM, Kurland LT. Seizure disorders in a Guamanian village. *Arch Neurol* 1962;**7**:37–44.

42 Mathai KV, Dunn DP, Kurland LT, Reeder FA. Convulsive disorders in the Mariana Islands. *Epilepsia* 1968;**9**:77–85.

43 Rose SW, Penry JK, Markush RE, Radloff LA, Putnam PL. Prevalence of epilepsy in children. *Epilepsia* 1973;**14**:133–52.

44. Rowan J, Hyman HH. The prevalence of epilepsy in a large heterogeneous urban population (The Bronx NY, Jan 8, 1975). *Trans American Neurol Assoc* 1976;**101**:281–3.

45 Meighan SS, Queener L, Weitman M. Prevalence of epilepsy in children of Multnomah County, Oregon. *Epilepsia* 1976;**17**:245–56.

46 Gomez JG, Arciniegas E, Torres J. Prevalence of epilepsy in Bogota, Colombia. *Neurology* 1978;**28**:90–5.

47 Chiofalo N, Kirschbaum EP, Fuentes A, Cordero M, Madsen J. Prevalence of epilepsy in children of Melipilla, Chile. *Epilepsia* 1979;**20**:261–6.

48 Gutierrez H, Rubio F, Escobedo F, Heron J. Prevalencia de epilepsia en ninos de edad escolar de una comunidad urbana de la Ciudad de Mexico. *Gaceta Medica Mexicana* 1980;**116**:497–501.

49 Beran RG, Hall L, Pesce A, *et al*. Population prevalence of epilepsy in Sydney, Australia. *Neuroepidemiology* 1982;**1**:201–8.

50 Osuntokun BO, Schoenberg BS, Nottidge VA, *et al*. Research protocol for measuring the prevalence of neurological disorders in developing countries. Results of a pilot study in Nigeria. *Neuroepidemiology* 1982;**1**:143–53.

51 Osuntokun BO, Adeuja AOG, Nottidge VA, et al. Prevalence of the epilepsies in Nigerian Africans: A community-based study. Epilepsia 1987;28:272–9.
52 Garcia-Pedroza F, Rubio-Donnadieu F, Garcia-Ramos G, et al. Prevalence of epilepsy in children: Tlalpan, Mexico City, Mexico. Neuroepidemiology 1983;2:16–23.
53 Proano J. Preliminary results of the neuroepidemiological study in Quiroga, Equador. Community Neurology (Quito) 1984;1:11–12.
54 Cruz M, Ruales J, Bossano F, et al. Estudios Neuroepidemiologicos en el Ecuador C.I.E.N. Fundacion Eugenio Espejo, Quito: Ministerio de Salud Publica, 1984.
55 Placencia M, Silva C, Cordova M, et al. Prevalencia de enfermedades neurologicas en una comunidad rural andina (Cangahua). Informe final, Quito: CONACYT 1984.
56 Kaamugisha J, Feksi AT. Determining the prevalence of epilepsy in the semi-urban population of Nakuru, Kenya, comparing two independent methods not apparently used before in epilepsy studies. Neuroepidemiology 1988;7:115–21.
57 Pradilla G, Pardo C, Puentes F, et al. Estudio neuroepidemiologico en Giron, Colombia. Comite de Neuroepidemiologia, Bucaramanga: Universidad Industrial de Santander, 1984.
58 Li SC, Schoenberg BS, Bolis CL, et al. Epidemiology of epilepsy in urban regions of the People's Republic of China. Epilepsia 1985;26:391-4.
59 Carpio A, Morales J, Calle H, Tinoco L, Santillan F. Prevalencia de epilepsia en la parroquia Cumbe, Azuay, Ecuador. Revista del Instituto de Ciencias de Salud Universidade de Cuenca (Ecuador) 1986;1:10–31.
60 Bharucha NE, Bharucha EP, Bharucha AE, Bhishe AV, Schoenberg BS. Prevalence of epilepsy in the Parsi community of Bombay. Epilepsia 1988;29:111–15.
61 Bondestam S, Garssen J, Abdulwakil A. Prevalence and treatment of mental disorders and epilepsy in Zanzibar. Acta Psychiat Scand 1990;81:327–31.
62 Tekle-Haimanot R, Forsgren L, Abebe M, et al. Clinical and electroencephalographic characteristics of epilepsy in rural Ethiopia: a community-based study. Epilepsy Res 1990;7:230–9.
63 Lavados J, Germain L, Morales A, et al. A descriptive study of epilepsy in the district of El Salvador, Chile. Acta Neurol Scand 1992;85:249–56.
64 Rwiza HT, Kilonzo GP, Haule J, et al. Prevalence and incidence of epilepsy in Ulanga, a rural district: a community-based study. Epilepsia 1992;33:1051–6.
65 Aziz H, Ali SM, Frances P, Khan MI, Hasan KZ. Epilepsy in Pakistan: a population-based epidemiological study. Epilepsia 1994;35:950–8.
66 Mendizabal JE, Salguero LF. Prevalence of epilepsy in a rural community of Guatemala. Epilepsia 1996;37:373–6.
67 Commission on classification and terminology of the International League of epilepsy. Proposal for revised clinical and electroencephalographic classification of epileptic seizures. Epilepsia 1981;22:489–501.
68 Lavy S, Carmon A, Yahr I. Assessment of clinical and electro-encephalographic classification of epileptic patients in everyday neurological practice. Epilepsia 1972;13:498–508.
69 Shorvon SD. The spectrum of epileptic seizures and syndromes. In: Duncan JS, Shorvon SD, Fish DR. eds. Clinical Epilepsy. Edinburgh: Churchill Livingstone 1995:25–101.
70 van Donselaar CA, Geerts AT, Meulstee J, Habbema JDF, Staal A. Reliability of the diagnosis of a first seizure. Neurology 1989;39:267–71.
71 Alter M, Masland RL, Kurtzke JF, Reed DM. Proposed definitions and classifications of epilepsy for epidemiological purposes. In: Alter M, Hauser WA. eds. The epidemiology of epilepsy: a workshop. Washington: NIH, NINDS monograph; chapter 27, 1972;147–48.

72 Sotelo J, Guerrero V, Rubio F. Neurocysticercosis: a new classification based on inactive and active forms. *Arch Inter Med* 1985;**145**:442–5.

73 Alarcon G, Olivares L. Cisticercosis Cerebral. Manifestaciones en un medio de alta prevalencia. *Revista de Investigaciones Clinicas* 1975;**27**:209–15.

74 Del Bruto OH, Santibanez R, Noboa CA, Aguirre R, Diaz E, Alarcon TA. Epilepsy due to neurocysticercosis: analysis of 203 patients. *Neurology* 1992;**42**:389–92.

75 Gastaut H, Gastaut JA, Gastaut JL, Roger J, Tassinari CA. Epilepsie Generalisee primarie. In: Lugaresi E, Pazzaglia P, Tassinari CA. eds. *Evolution and Prognosis of the epilepsies*. Bologna: Aulo Gaggi, 1973;23–35.

76 Commission on classification and terminology of the International League of epilepsy. Proposal for revised international classification of epilepsies, epileptic syndromes and related seizure disorders. *Epilepsia* 1989; **30**:389–99.

77 Manford M, Hart YM, Sander JWAS, Shorvon SD. The National General practice study of epilepsy: The syndromic classification of the ILAE applied to epilepsy in a general population. *Arch Neurol* 1992;**49**:801–8.

78 Commission of Epidemiology and Prognosis. Guidelines for Epidemiological Studies on Epilepsy. *Epilepsia* 1993;**34**:592–6.

79 Annegers JF, Hauser WA, Elveback LR. Remission of seizures and relapse in patients with epilepsy. *Epilepsy* 1979;**20**:729–37.

80 Lennox W. *Epilepsy and Related Disorders.* London: Churchill, 1960.

81 Quirk JA, Fish DR, Smith SJM, Sander JWAS, Shorvon SD, Allen PJ. Incidence of photosensitive epileptic seizures: a prospective national study. *Electroenceph Clin Neurophysiol* 1995;**95**:260–7.

82 Sato S. The epidemiological and clinico-statistical study of epilepsy in Nigata City. *Clinical Neurology* (Tokio) 1964;**4**:413–24.

83 Forsgren L, Bucht G, Eriksson S, Bergmark L. Incidence and clinical characterization of unprovoked seizures in adults—a prospective population-based study. *Epilepsia* 1996;**37**:224–9.

84 Miller FJW, Court SDM, Walton WS, Know EG. *Growing up in Newcastle-upon-Tyne. A Continuing Study of Health and Illness in Young Children with their Families.* London: Oxford University Press, 1960.

85 Crombie DL, Cross KW, Fry J, *et al.* A survey of the epilepsies in general practice. A report by the Research Committee of the College of General Practitioners. *BMJ* 1960;**ii**:416–22.

86 Levy LF, Forbes Jl, Parirenyatwa TS. Epilepsy in Africans. *Central Africa Journal of Medicine* 1964;**10**:241–9.

87 Jilek-Aall L. Epilepsy in the Wapogoro tribe in Tanganyka. *Acta Psychiat Scand* 1965;**41**:57–86.

88 Dada T. Epilepsy in Lagos, Nigeria. *African Journal of Medicine* 1970; **1**:161–84.

89 Poskanzer DC. A house-to-house survey of a community for epilepsy. In: Milton A, Hauser WA. eds. *The epidemiology of epilepsy: a workshop.* NINDS Monograph no. 14. Washington: DHEW. 1972:45–6.

90 Baumann RJ, Marx MB, Leonidakis MG. An estimate of the prevalence of epilepsy in a rural Appalachian population. *Am J Epidem* 1977;**106**:45–52.

91 Baumann R, Marx M, Leonidakis M. Epilepsy in Rural Kentucky: Prevalence in a population of school age children. *Epilepsia* 1978;**19**:75–80.

92 Pascual M, Pascual J, Rodriguez L, Rojas F, Tejeiros A. La epilepsia: estudio epidemiologico en una poblacion infantil. *Bol Medico Hospital Infantil Mexico* 1980;**37**:811–21.

93 Goudsmit J, van der Waals FW, Gajdusek DC. Epilepsy in the Gbawein and Wroughbarth Clan of Gran Bassa County, Liberia: the endemic occurrence of "See-ee" in the native population. *Neuroepidemiology* 1983;**2**:24–34.

94 Ponce P, Fernandez R, D'Souse C, et al. Estudio de prevalencia de transtornos neurologicos en Lezama. In: Ponce P. (ed). Estudios neuroepidemiologicos in Venezuela. Departamento de Enfermedades Neurologicas. Caracas: Ministerio de Sanidad y Asistencia Social; 1985:16–38.

95 Haerer AF, Anderson DW, Schoenberg BS. Prevalence and clinical features of epilepsy in a biracial United States population. Epilepsia 1986;27:66–75.

96 Joensen P. Prevalence, incidence and classification of epilepsy in the Faroes. Acta Neurol Scand 1986;74:150–5.

97 Marino Jr R, Cukiert A, Pinho E. Epidemiological aspects of epilepsy in S. Paulo, Brazil. In: Wolf P, Dam M, Dreifuss FE. (eds). Advances in Epileptology – XVIth Epilepsy International Symposium. New York: Raven Press 1987.

98 Koul R et al. Prevalence and pattern of epilepsy (Lath/Mirgi/Laran) in Rural Kashmir, India. Epilepsia 1988;29:116–22.

99 Zuloaga L, Soto C, Jaramilo D. Prevalencia de epilepsia en la ciudad de Medellin. Boletin OPS 1988;104:331–4.

100 Tsuboi T. Prevalence and incidence of epilepsy in Tokio. Epilepsia 1988;29:103–10.

101 Cowan L, Bodensteiner JB, Leviton A, Doherty L. Prevalence of the epilepsies in children and adolescents. Epilepsia 1989;30:94–106.

102 Chiofalo N, Schoenberg BS, Kirschbaum A, et al. Estudios epidemiologicos de las enfermedades neurologicas en Santiago Metropolitano, Chile. Abstracts of the IV Pan American Congress of Neuroepidemiology. Cartagena, Colombia, 1989; 17–18

103 Bird AV, Heinz HJ, Klintworth PG. Convulsive disorders in Bantu mineworkers. Epilepsia 1962;3:175–87.

104 Baumann RJ. Classification and population studies of epilepsy. In: Anderson VE, Hauser WA, Penry JK, Singh CF. eds. Genetic basis of the epilepsies. New York: Raven Press 1982:11–20

105 Delacourt A, Breteler MMB, Meinardi H, Hauser WA, Hofman A. Prevalence of epilepsy in the elderly—the Rotterdam Study. Epilepsia 1996;37:141–7.

106 Van den Berg BJ, Yeruhalmy J. Studies on convulsive disorders in young children. 1. Incidence of febrile and nonfebrile convulsions by age and other factors. Pediatr Res 1969;3:298–304.

107 Jilek-Aall L, Jilek W, Miller JR. Clinical and genetic aspects of seizure disorders prevalent in an isolated African Population. Epilepsia 1979;20:613–22.

108 Fernandez JG, Schmidt MI, Tozzi S, Sander JWAS. Prevalence of epilepsy: the Porto Alegre study. Epilepsia 1992;33(S3):132.

109 Gracia F, Lao SL, Castillo L, et al. Epidemiology of epilepsy in Guayami Indians from Boca del Toro Province, Republic of Panama. Epilepsia 1990;31:718–23.

110 Hauser WA, Hesdorffer DC. Epilepsy: frequency, causes and consequences. Maryland: Demos Publications, 1990.

111 Nashef L, Sander JWAS, Shorvon SD. The Mortality of Epilepsy. In: Pedley TA, Meldrum BS. eds. Recent Advances in Epilepsy—Volume 6. Edinburgh: Churchill Livingstone; 1995;271–87.

112 Sander JWAS. The prognosis, morbidity and mortality of epilepsy. In: Duncan JS, Shorvon SD, Fish DR. eds. Clinical Epilepsy. Edinburgh: Churchill Livingstone; 1995;300–20.

113 Cockerell OC, Johnson AL, Sander JWAS, Shorvon SD. The mortality of early epilepsy: the results of a community based study. Lancet 1994;344:918–21.

114 Klenerman P, Sander JWAS, Shorvon SD. Mortality of epilepsy: a study in patients in long term residential care. J Neurol Neurosurg Psychiat 1993;56:149–52.

115 Nashef L, Fish D, Sander JWAS, Shorvon SD. Incidence of sudden unexpected death in an outpatient cohort with epilepsy at a tertiary referral centre. *J Neurol Neurosurg Psychiat* 1995;**58**:462–4.

116 Placencia M, Sander JWAS, Roman M, *et al*. The characteristics of epilepsy in a largely untreated population in Rural Ecuador. *J Neurol Neurosurg Psychiat* 1994;**57**:320–5.

117 Sander JWAS, Hart YM, Johnson AL, Shorvon SD. Seizures in childhood: a prospective community based cohort study. *Acta Neurol Scand* 1990;**82**:S9.

118 Sander JWAS, Cockerell OC, Hart YM, Shorvon SD. Is the incidence of epilepsy falling in the UK? *Lancet* 1993;**342**:874.

119 Hart YM, Shorvon SD. The nature of epilepsy in the general population. I. Characteristics of patients receiving medication for epilepsy. *Epilepsy Res* 1995;**21**:43–9.

120 Li LM, Fish DR, Sisodiya SM, Shorvon SD, Alsanjari N, Stevens JM. High resolution magnetic resonance imaging in adults with partial or secondary generalised epilepsy attending a tertiary referral unit. *J Neurol Neurosurg Psychiat* 1995;**59**:384–7.

121 Annegers JF, Grabow JD, Groover RV, *et al*. Seizures after head trauma: a population study. *Neurology* 1980;**30**:683–39.

122 Jennett B. Epidemiology of head injury. *J Neurol Neurosurg Psychiat* 1996;**60**:362–9.

123 Morrell DC, Gage HG, Robinson NA. Symptoms in general practice. *J R Gen Pract* 1971;**21**:32–43.

124 Nelson KB, Ellenberg JH. Predictors of epilepsy in children who have experienced febrile seizures. *N Engl J Med* 1976;**295**:1029–33.

125 Kurtzke JR. Mortality and morbidity data on epilepsy. In: Alter M. and Hauser WA. eds. *The Epidemiology of Epilepsy: a workshop*. NINDS monograph 14. Washington: DHEW 1972;21–36.

126 Wise PH, Kotelchuck M, Wilson ML, Mills M. Racial and socio-economic disparities in childhood mortality in Boston. *N Engl J Med* 1985;**313**:360–6.

127 National Health Survey. *Prevalence of Chronic Conditions in the United States*. Series 10 no. 109 (HRA no. 77–1536). Washington: DHWE, 1973.

128 Walker MC, Sander JWAS. The impact of new antiepileptic drugs in the prognosis of epilepsy: seizure freedom should be the ultimate goal. *Neurology* 1996;**46**:912–14.

129 Bittencourt PRM, Gracia CM, Lorenzana P. Epilepsy and parasitosis of the central nervous system. In: Pedley TA, Meldrum BS. eds. *Recent Advances in Epilepsy—Volume 3*. Edinburgh: Churchill Livingstone 1988;123–59.

130 Commission on Tropical diseases of the International League against epilepsy. Relationship between epilepsy and tropical diseases. *Epilepsia* 1994;**35**:89–93.

131 Schenone H, Ramirez R, Rojas A. Aspectos epidemiologicos de la neurocistercercoses en Latino–America. *Boletim Chileno de Parasitologia* 1973; **28**:61–72.

132 Sakamoto A. *Estudo clinico e prognostico das crises epilepticas que iniciam na infancia numa populacao brasileira*. Tese de doutorado, Universidade de Sao Paulo (Ribeirao Preto) 1985.

133 Arruda WO. Etiology of epilepsy. A prospective study of 200 cases. *Arq Neuropsiquiat* 1991;**49**:251–4.

134 Garcia HH, Gilman R, Martinez M *et al*. Cysticercosis as a major cause of epilepsy in Peru. *Lancet* 1993;**341**:197–200.

135 Cruz ME, Barry M, Cruz R, *et al*. Prevalence of neurocysticercosis in an Andean community in Ecuador. *Neuroepidemiology* 1995;**14**:29.

136 Senanayake N, Roman G. Aetiological factors of epilepsy in the tropics. *J Trop Geo Neurol* 1991;**1**:69–80.

163

137 Senanayake N, Roman G. Epidemiology of epilepsy in the tropics. *J Trop Geo Neurol* 1992;2:610–19.
138 Pitella JEH. Lana MA. Brain involvement in hepatosplenic Schistosomiasis mansoni. *Brain* 1981;**104**:621–32.
139 Jardim E, Takayanagui OM. Epilepsia e doenca de Chagas cronica. *Arq Neuropsiquiat* 1981;**39**:32–41
140 Raymond AA, Fish DR, Stevens JM, Cook MJ, Sisodiya SM, Shorvon SD. Subependimal heterotopia: a distinct neuronal migration defect associated with epilepsy. *J Neurol Neurosurg Psychiat* 1994;**57**:1195–202.
141 Raymond AA, Fish DR, Stevens JM, Sisodiya SM, Shorvon SD. Abnormalities of gyration, heterotopias, focal cortical dysplasias, micro-dysgenesis, dysembryoplastic neuroepithelial tumour and dysgenesis of the archicortex in epilepsy. Clinical, electroencephalographic and neuroimaging features in 100 adult patients. *Brain* 1995;**118**:629–60.
142 Shorvon SD. *Status epilepticus: its clinical features and treatment in children and adults.* Cambridge University Press 1994;304–5.
143 Scheffer IE, Bhatia KP, Lopes-Cendes I, *et al.* Autosomal dominant frontal lobe epilepsy misdiagnosed as sleep disorder. *Lancet* 1994;**343**:515–17.
144 Simard JM, Garcia-Bengochea F, Ballinger WE, Mickle JP, Quisling RG. Cavernous angioma: a review of 126 collected and 12 new clinical cases. *Neurosurgery* 1986;**18**:162–72.

Appendix 1: ILAE Guidelines for epidemiologic studies (Adapted from reference 78)

1. Definitions

Epileptic seizure A clinical manifestation presumed to result from an abnormal and excessive discharge of a set of neurons in the brain. The clinical manifestation consists of sudden and transitory abnormal phenomena which may include alterations of consciousness, motorsensory, autonomic, or psychic events, perceived by the patient or an observer.

Epilepsy A condition characterised by recurrent (two or more) epileptic seizures, unprovoked by any immediate identified cause. Multiple seizures occurring in a 24 hour period are considered a single event. An episode of status epilepticus is considered a single event. Individuals who have had only febrile seizures or only neonatal seizures as herein defined are excluded from this category.

Status epilepticus A single epileptic seizure of >30-min duration or a series of epileptic seizures during which function is not regained between ictal events in a >30-min period.

"Active epilepsy" A prevalent case of active epilepsy is defined as a person with epilepsy who has had at least one epileptic seizure in the previous five years, regardless of antiepileptic drug (AED) treatment. A case under treatment is someone with the diagnosis of epilepsy receiving (or having received) AEDs on prevalence day.

Epilepsy in remission with treatment A prevalent case of epilepsy with no seizures for five or more years and receiving AEDs at the time of ascertainment.

Epilepsy in remission without treatment A prevalent case of epilepsy with no seizures for five or more years and not receiving AEDs at the time of ascertainment.

Single or isolated seizure One or more epileptic seizures occurring in a period of 24 hours.

Febrile seizure An epileptic seizure as herein defined, occurring in childhood after age 1 month associated with a febrile illness not caused by an infection of the CNS, without previous neonatal seizures or a previous unprovoked seizure, and not meeting criteria for other acute symptomatic seizures.

Neonatal seizure An epileptic seizure as herein defined occurring in the first four weeks of life.

Febrile seizure with neonatal seizure One or more neonatal seizures in a child who has also experienced one or more febrile seizures as herein defined.

Nonepileptic events Clinical manifestations presumed to be unrelated to an abnormal and excessive discharge of a set of neurons of the brain, including: (a) disturbances in the brain function (vertigo or dizziness, syncope, sleep and movement disorders, transient global amnesia, migraine, enuresis), and (b) pseudoseizures (nonepileptic sudden behavioural episodes presumed to be of psychogenic origin; these may coexist with true epileptic seizures).

165

2. Seizure type classification

2.1 Generalised seizures A seizure is considered generalised when clinical symptomatology provides no indication of an anatomic localisation and no clinical evidence of focal onset. When possible, three main seizures subtypes may be categorised:

Generalised convulsive seizures with predominantly tonic, atonic, clonic, or tonic-clonic features

Generalised nonconvulsive seizures represented by absence seizure

Myoclonic seizures

In patients who have experienced several types of generalised seizure each seizure type must be categorised.

2.2 Partial seizures A seizure should be classified as partial when there is evidence of a clinical partial onset, regardless of whether the seizure is secondarily generalised. The first clinical signs of a seizure ("the aura"), have a highly localising value and result from the anatomic or functional neuronal activation of part of one hemisphere.

When alertness and ability to interact appropriately with the environment is maintained, the seizure is classified as a simple partial seizure.

When impairment of consciousness, amnesia, or confusion during or after a seizure is reported, the seizure is classified as a complex partial seizure.

When a seizure becomes secondarily generalised, the seizure is classified as partial seizure, secondarily generalised (simple or complex).

When the distinction between simple and complex partial seizure cannot be made, from information provided by history and medical records, the seizure is classified as partial epileptic seizure of unknown type.

When a patient has several types of partial seizure, each should be separately categorised.

2.3 Multiple seizure type When both generalised and partial seizures are associated, each type must be described.

2.4 Unclassified seizures The term unclassified seizures should be used when it is impossible to classify seizures owing to lack of adequate information.

3. Aetiology and risk factors

Epileptic seizures and the epilepsies may be a manifestation of many cerebral or systemic diseases. The first step in categorisation of seizures should be based on the presence or absence of a presumed acute precipitating insult, which will permit distinction into provoked or unprovoked seizures. Single or recurrent unprovoked seizures may belong to two possible categories: symptomatic seizures or epilepsies and seizures or epilepsies of unknown cause.

3.1 Symptomatic seizures or epilepsies are considered to be the consequence of a known or suspected cerebral dysfunction.

3.1.1 *Provoked seizures* (acute symptomatic seizures): Seizure(s) occurring in close temporal association with an acute systemic, metabolic, or toxic insult or in association with an acute CNS insult (infection, stroke, cranial trauma, intracerebral haemorrhage, or acute alcohol intoxication or withdrawal). Such seizures are often isolated epileptic events associated with acute conditions, but may also be recurrent seizures or even status epilepticus when the acute conditions recurs, e.g. in alcohol withdrawal seizures.

3.1.2 *Unprovoked seizures*: Seizures may occur in relation to a well demonstrated antecedent condition, substantially increasing the risk for epileptic seizures. Two major subgroups may be categorised:

(i) Remote symptomatic unprovoked seizures owing to conditions resulting in a static encephalopathy. Such cases are individuals with epilepsy subsequent to an insult of the CNS, such as infection, cerebral trauma, or cerebrovascular disease, which are generally presumed to result in a non-progressive (static) lesion.

(ii) Symptomatic unprovoked seizures owing to progressive CNS disorders.

3.2 Unprovoked seizures of unknown aetiology: Cases of unprovoked seizures for which no clear antecedent aetiology can be detected. If possible, these cases can be further classified into the following subheadings:

3.2.1 *Idiopathic epilepsies:* The term idiopathic is used here as defined by the ILAE[76] and must be reserved for certain partial or generalised epileptic syndromes with particular clinical characteristics and with specific EEG finding, and should not be generally used to refer to epilepsy or seizures without obvious cause.

3.2.2 *Cryptogenic epilepsies:* The term cryptogenic is used to include partial or generalised unprovoked seizures or epilepsies in which no factor associated with increased risk of seizures has been identified. This group includes patients who do not conform to the criteria for the symptomatic or idiopathic categories. Whenever possible, the Commission on Epidemiology and Prognosis encourages use of the most recent ILAE Classification of Epilepsies and Epileptic Syndromes.[76] Appropriate categorisation of individual cases may require use of state of the art technologies and procedures. In many settings in which epidemiologic studies are conducted, in particular in field situations, all required information for proper classification of epileptic syndromes cannot be obtained.

8 Amyotrophic lateral sclerosis

GUSTAVO ROMÁN

> - There is surprisingly little geographical variation in the incidence of amyotrophic lateral sclerosis.
> - Mortality from amyotrophic lateral sclerosis is increasing over time in many countries. Whether this reflects an underlying increase in incidence is not known.
> - In the Guamanian form of the disease both genetic predisposition and environmental neurotoxins are implicated in aetiology.
> - The relevance of the Guamanian form of amyotrophic lateral sclerosis to amyotrophic lateral sclerosis generally is still unclear.

J M Charcot, at La Salpêtrière Hospital in Paris, first identified amyotrophic lateral sclerosis (ALS) from among the heterogeneous group of the spinal muscular atrophies. Between 1872 and 1874, in his *Lectures on the diseases of the nervous system* (lectures XII and XIII), Charcot masterfully described the clinical and anatomopathological features of the disease that bears his name (*Maladie de Charcot*).[1] The growing complexity of this field is reflected in the current classification of the spinal muscular atrophies and other disorders of the motor neurons prepared by the World Federation of Neurology (WFN) Research Group on Neuromuscular Disorders.[2] Likewise, the difficulties in clinically separating cases of ALS from other related forms of the disease for epidemiological studies, for clinical research, and for therapeutic trials, led to the successful meeting in El Escorial, Spain, of a group of experts under the aegis of the WFN to define precise criteria for the clinical, electrophysiological, and neuropathological diagnosis of ALS.[3] El Escorial WFN criteria have been recently validated,[4] and offer a solid foundation for future epidemiological studies of ALS.

Case definition

El Escorial WFN criteria for the diagnosis of ALS require the presence of signs of lower and upper motor neuron damage on clinical examination, and progressive spread of these signs within a region or to other regions, in the absence of electrophysiological and neuroimaging evidence of other disease processes that might explain the clinical signs. Repetition of clinical examination at least every six months is required to assess progression of the disease.

These criteria are stratified clinically in four levels of diagnostic certainty: *definite, probable, possible,* and *suspected ALS.* Also, the criteria allow for inclusion of several forms of ALS that present with various other clinical features, or particular genetic or epidemiological characteristics. These include the following types: *sporadic ALS*—the classic form of the disease, *coexistent-sporadic ALS,* the *ALS related syndromes,* and *ALS-variants.* The last two have provided some of the most interesting clues to the pathogenesis of ALS.

Descriptive epidemiology

It must be mentioned at the outset that, with few exceptions, most epidemiological studies of ALS failed to separate this condition from other forms of motor neuron disease. This was due in part to the absence, until recently, of diagnostic criteria for ALS, and to the fact that even in the latest neurological adaptation of the 10th International Classification of Diseases (ICD-10 NA),[5] the major sporadic motor neuron diseases of adults (including ALS, progressive spinal muscular atrophy, progressive bulbar palsy, and mixed forms) are coded under a single category (G12·2: disorders of motor neuron of undetermined aetiology). Thus, ALS represents most cases of motor neuron disease in all series (about 80%–90%) and failure to separate other conditions may introduce a 10% error in incidence data and a larger one in prevalence data.[6] Furthermore, difficulties with clinical diagnoses, incomplete case ascertainment, and subreporting, all adversely affect epidemiological data on ALS.

Incidence, prevalence, mortality

The above caveats notwithstanding, a relatively narrow margin of incidence and prevalence for motor neuron disease has been reported in most of the world (table 8.1).

Incidence

Chancellor and Warlow[7] have recently published a useful review of incidence of motor neuron disease worldwide. The average crude incidence rates for motor neuron disease in several countries ranged from 0·4 to 2·6/100 000/year.[6-9] Annual incidence rates for ALS ranged from 0·6 to 1·5/100 000. It is unclear if incidence rates of motor neuron disease lower than 1/100 000/year represent true low disease incidence or limitations in case ascertainment. Most studies showed a trend towards increasing age specific incidence rates with advancing age, beginning at about age 50–59 and reaching a peak at 75 years of age, to decrease again to lower rates at the age of 80 and older. In most studies, motor neuron disease predominated in males, with reported men to women ratios ranging from 1·2:1 to 2·6:1. It has been hypothesised that this male preponderance could be the result of hormone influences or a confounder for putative risk factors such as trauma, occupational exposure, and physical activity.[6] However, it has also been suggested that the lower ALS rates reported for elderly women may result from incomplete case ascertainment.[9]

Prevalence

Crude prevalence ratios for motor neuron disease showed, in general, a wider range than those for incidence, ranging from 0·8 to 8·5 per 100 000 (table 8.1). As in the case of incidence, prevalence ratios lower than 1·5/100 000 may represent regions of lower risk but also raise issues of limitations in case ascertainment, methodological differences, and variations in the reference point for prevalence data, as these diseases have short survival times. Quality of medical care is also reflected in longer survival times and higher prevalence figures. Reported patterns for age and sex specific prevalence seem to be similar to those for incidence.

170

Table 8.1 Worldwide incidence and prevalence of motor neuron disease*

Geographic areas	Study period	Incidence†	Prevalence‡
Europe:			
Iceland	1954–63	0·8	6·4
Norway	1974–75	2·1	
Sweden	1970–81	2·6	4·8–8·5
Finland	1976–81	2·4	2·4–8·4
Denmark	1974–86	1·5	2·5
Russia	1963–70		3·7
Germany	1941–55		2·5
England and Wales	1981	2·2	7·0
Switzerland	1951–67	1·7	6·7
Poland	1964	0·8	2·2
Rumania	1950–52		3·7
France	1986–87	1·3	7·7
Italy (several studies)	1964–85	0·6–1·9	1·6–2·6
Spain	1974–85	1·0	3·5
America:			
Canada (several studies)	1978–84	0·9–2·4	4·9
Unites States (several studies)	1925–84	1·2–2·4	6·4
Mexico	1962–69	0·4	0·8
Africa:			
Israel (several studies)	1959–74	0·5–0·8	3·0
Tunisia	1974–80	0·45	
Libya	1980–85	0·87	3·4
Asia:			
China (several studies)	1983–85		4·5–7·9
India	1982–84		4·0
Japan (except Kii peninsula)	1954–72		1·5–5·8
Japan (Kii peninsula)	1957–72	55·0	96·9–194·3§
Oceania:			
Hawaii	1952–69	1·0	
Guam	1944–85	179·0–12·0§	
Western New Guinea	1975–80	147·0	1300·0

* Modified from data previously summarised.[6-9]
† Average crude incidence rates/100 000/year.
‡ Average crude prevalence ratios/100 000.
§ Adjusted to the 1970 United States population.

Mortality

Mortality data from death certificates are readily available and could allow for comparisons of disease frequency. However, there are wide variations in international mortality rates for motor neuron disease, probably representing both differences in quality of the death certificates (subreporting at time of death), failure to clinically identify the disease of interest, and differences in methodology.[10]

In industrialised countries, identification of patients with motor neuron disease from death certificates seems to be reasonably accurate (72 and 96% of the cases).[11-13] None the less, even within industrialised nations, considerable variation in average age adjusted mortality for motor neuron disease has been reported (for ages 40 and over per 100 000 per year), as follows: Sweden (1960–90)[14] 3·81, Ireland (1978–87)[15] 3·38, USA (1971, 1973–78)[16] 2·61, England and Wales (1963–89)[15 17] 2·60, Finland

(1963–72)[18] 2·35, France (1968–90)[19] 2·13, and Italy (1958–87)[20] 1·51.

Studies of the time trends for mortality from motor neuron disease have shown a tendency towards longitudinal increase in mortality in several countries, particularly in Sweden,[14] Ireland,[15] England and Wales,[17] France,[19] Italy,[20] Norway,[21] Japan,[22] and the USA.[23] This trend has been explained by several factors including better knowledge of the disease among physicians, increased numbers of neurologists, and the so-called Gompertzian effect, or inter-disease competition, whereby better survival from high mortality conditions in old age (stroke and heart disease) would allow the expression of the disease in surviving older patients.[14 17 19 21 22 24] An increase in mortality rates for Parkinson's disease, another neurological disease of elderly people, has also been reported since the 1950s probably as a reflection of increase in the susceptible aged population.[25]

Analytical epidemiology

Risk factors

In a similar manner to Parkinson's disease,[25] the unknown duration of the incubation period for ALS and the uncertainty of the relevant exposures preclude long term prospective studies comparing exposed and unexposed cohorts. The low frequency of ALS, as well as recall bias, limit case-control studies with appropriate statistical power. Thus no clearly defined risk factors for ALS have been identified.

Case-control studies comparing urban and rural populations in Italy[26 27] found increased risk for ALS among rural populations of lower sociocultural level, and in occupations involving manual labour and physical activity, mainly farmers (which may indicate exposure to neurotoxic products used in agriculture) and handlers of animal hides or carcasses (a possible surrogate for zoonotic infections, including retroviruses). Also, in community based surveys of motor neuron disease an increased risk has been found in rural populations—reflected in two to seven times more cases found in the agricultural and farmworking populations.[28–32] Other less well defined risk factors include exposure to chemical solvents, electrical fields and welding, heavy metals, alcohol consumption, and smoking.[7–9]

Clusters

Small clusters of non-familial adult onset motor neuron disease have been reported, including cases living in the same block,[33][34] having similar occupations,[35][36] or with time clustering of disease onset within a small United States community.[37] In the last, probable chemical exposure was found either from consumption of freshly caught Lake Michigan fish (five of six cases) or from occupational use of chemicals (two of six cases). Analysis of another perceived cluster of nine cases in a United States community showed this to be a random event.[38]

An apparent epidemic cluster of motor neuron disease has been described in Sweden, occurring among men living in the county of Skaraborg between 1973 and 1984.[39][40] Based initially on analysis of death certificates for Sweden in the period 1961–90,[39] the study then actively searched all cases of motor neuron disease in this community and compared the results with those of the adjacent county of Värmland.[40] During the period 1973–84, an epidemic-like increase in cases among older men was found with an average annual incidence of 4/100 000 person-years (70 males identified), compared with an incidence of 2·8 for males and 1·6 for females during the entire period 1961–90. These patients were found to have higher age at onset of motor neuron disease and more frequent than expected employment in agriculture.[40]

Based on these results, an extensive case-control study of motor neuron disease was performed,[41] showing that the highest odds ratio (OR) for the disease (OR = 15–18, lower limit 95% confidence interval (95% CI) 2·8) corresponded to the combination of heredity (family history of neurodegenerative or thyroid disease), male sex, and exposure to solvents. On the basis of these studies, Gunnarsson[42] postulated that motor neuron disease may occur in a genetically susceptible population subset. These people may have defective detoxification leading to the neurodegenerative process precipitated by different agents after an induction period of one to two decades.[14][42]

Trauma

"Lou Gehrig's disease" identifies ALS in the United States after the famous New York baseball player who died in 1941, aged 37, of this disease. Some case-control studies have found increased risk associated with physical activity, as well as with previous mechanical, chemical, surgical, and electrical trauma.[7-9] However, no safe inferences can be drawn from most of these studies. The evidence in favour of previous remote trauma as a risk factor for ALS has been recently reviewed,[43] only to be strongly criticised and basically disallowed due to serious methodological shortcomings.[44]

Aetiological studies

By contrast with the largely inconclusive results of analytical epidemiology, some clinical observations included in the group of the *ALS related syndromes* and *ALS-variants* have provided important information. Among those explored are the *ALS related syndromes* occurring in association with toxins (heavy metals, organic pesticides),[3] endocrine disorders (hyperthyroidism, hyperparathyroidism, hypogonadism, etc),[3] immune or lymphoproliferative disorders,[45 46] and infections, in particular polio,[47 48] and retroviruses such as HTLV-I,[49-51] found with high prevalence in some areas of Japan, the Caribbean, and Latin America.

The *familial ALS (FALS)-variants* have also contributed to the pathogenesis of ALS. Recently, patients with chromosome 21 associated FALS were found to possess dominantly inherited mutations in the gene that encodes copper-zinc superoxide dismutase (CuZnSOD).[52] This enzyme defect resulted in high catalytic activity of the peroxidase reaction, inducing in cell cultures H_2O_2 mediated apoptosis or programmed neuronal death which could be inhibited by copper chelators, offering a novel therapeutic approach with chelators and antioxidants.[52]

Demonstration of abnormally high concentrations of glutamate and aspartate in plasma and CSF of patients with ALS,[53-56] led to subsequent research on excitotoxicity—that is, the effect of excitatory amino acid neurotransmitters on neuronal death in neurodegenerative diseases.[57] Controlled clinical trials of riluzole,[58] an agent that alters glutamate release and protects against glutamate toxicity, resulted in its recent approval for treatment of ALS.

Geographic aspects

Geographic variants

Peculiar geographic ALS-variants include early onset forms of ALS. The *Madras form*, described in India, begins between 10 and

30 years of age and is characterised by bulbopontine involvement, distal atrophy of the limbs, deafness, and a chronic benign course.[59] It resembles the chromosome 2 associated juvenile FALS form described in Tunisia.[60] These variants provide evidence in favour of the clinical and genetic heterogeneity of ALS.

Geographic isolates

The extraordinary frequency of ALS and parkinsonism-dementia complex in remote areas of the western Pacific remains an intensively studied but as yet unsolved major problem in neuroepidemiology. These high incidence geographic isolates occur in the Mariana Islands—mainly Guam and Rota,[61-64] the Kii peninsula of Japan,[65] and the west Irian region of New Guinea,[66] resulting in rates of incidence, prevalence, and mortality 50 to 100 times larger than those found elsewhere in the world (table 8.1).

Guamanian motor neuron disease

In 1956, the United States National Institute of Neurological Disorders and Stroke (NINDS) established on Guam a registry for cases of motor neuron disease and parkinsonism-dementia complex. Originals are kept locally, but complete copies of medical records, death certificates, and epidemiological and pathology reports were deposited and inventoried at the Neuroepidemiology Branch, NINDS, National Institutes of Health in Bethesda, Maryland. Using this case registry, we analysed the epidemiological temporal pattern of occurrence of motor neuron disease on Guam from 1941 to 1985, to define the duration of the latency period for the disease, the most recent years of meaningful risk, and the critical age for acquiring the disease.[67] Likewise, we investigated the geographic occurrence at onset of disease,[68] using election districts—the smallest defined areas with population information available from 1956 to the end of 1985.

Chamorro family histories were traced taking into account that Guam was a Spanish colony until 1899 and, therefore, married Chamorro women follow the complex surnames customs used in Spain. This factor could have influenced previous efforts to find a familial pattern of inheritance on Guam.[69 70]

Finally, we undertook a correlation analysis to investigate the relation between these demographic, geographic, and familial data with elements of the two main causal hypotheses—that is, cycad neurotoxins[71] and mineral content (low calcium, high aluminium) in water and soil.[72]

Epidemiology of guamanian motor neuron disease

A group of 407 Chamorros with motor neuron disease (255 men (63%) and 152 women) were included in the analysis; in 171 (44%) the diagnosis was confirmed by pathology. The men to women ratio was 2·2. The median age at onset was 48 (range 19–84) years with a median duration of the disease from onset to death of about 4 (range 0·2–24·8) years. Average *age adjusted annual incidence rates* peaked at 179/100 000 for men in 1959–61 and 61/100 000 for women in 1956–58. Since then, a steady downward pattern has occurred (figure 8.1). From 1941 to the end of 1985, the median age at onset increased for both sexes (from 42 to 56 years for men, and from 42 to 55 years for women) but the men to women ratio declined from 2·5 to 1·5.

We calculated the observed to expected ratios for number of cases of motor neuron disease occurring in birth cohorts from

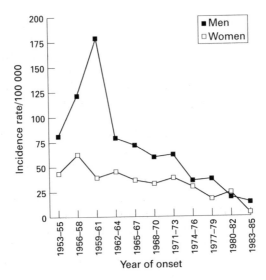

Figure 8.1   Average annual age adjusted incidence rates, by sex, for Chamorros with onset of motor neuron disease on Guam: three year periods, 1956–85 (from Zhang et al[67] with permission).

1886 to the end of 1950. The ratios peaked for both sexes in those born between 1901 and 1910 and declined in the birth cohorts after 1930–35. By the end of 1987 no Chamorro born after 1949 had developed motor neuron disease.

The latency (or incubation) *period* is defined as the time interval between acquisition and onset of motor neuron disease and was inferred based on analysis of cases in migrants to and from Guam who subsequently developed motor neuron disease. The longest period was 34 years, found in a Chamorro born on Guam who resided overseas for that length of time, returned to Guam, and then developed motor neuron disease. The shortest incubation period was three years, found in a Filipino who lived in Guam 36 months before onset of motor neuron disease. In general, over time the exposure period on Guam to acquire motor neuron disease has increased, or the latent period has increased, or both have increased.[67]

In view of the clear decline of incidence of motor neuron disease on Guam, we analysed the most *recent years of meaningful risk for acquiring motor neuron disease*, based on migrants to Guam. There were six Filipino men and three United States white men who arrived on the island in the late 1940s (seven), 1956 (one), and 1963 (one) and developed motor neuron disease. Despite a large Filipino migration to Guam since 1960 no new cases of motor neuron disease have occurred in these migrants. Likewise, among Chamorro migrants who left Guam between 1934 and 1966 there were 41 cases of motor neuron disease, by contrast with only six cases of the disease among later migrants, despite a much larger emigration after 1966. Thus 1960 to 1966 seem to be the most recent years of meaningful risk for acquiring motor neuron disease on Guam.

We were also able to calculate the *critical age of exposure* for acquiring the disease on Guam. Based on data from Chamorro migrants, high risk exposure only in childhood failed to cause motor neuron disease, whereas high risk exposure during adolescence led to all the known cases. During the years of meaningful risk three to 10 years of exposure during adulthood may have led to development of motor neuron disease among some non-Chamorro migrants to Guam. The recent increase in latent or exposure periods and the decline in incidence could indicate a possible dose-response relation (lower levels of exposure to causative agents would result in longer latency periods).

Geographic distribution of guamanian motor neuron disease

Familial aggregation notwithstanding, we categorised the Guam districts as high, medium, and low risk areas. The two southern districts of Inarajan and Umatac showed average annual age adjusted incidence rates of motor neuron disease that were significantly higher than the overall rate. Geographic patterns of incidence were significantly related to the number of persons per household (Spearman rank correlation coefficient $(r) = 0.64$), median income per family ($r = -0.52$), and years of education ($r = -0.48$), indicating (for men only) higher incidence in lower socioeconomic groups.

Over time, high incidence of motor neuron disease persisted longer in these same southern districts, especially for men. This has been attributed in part to the geographical isolation and poverty of this region, particularly in Umatac. By contrast with central districts of Guam where economic development and westernisation advanced more rapidly after the end of the second world war, the south retained longer a subsistence economy and a traditional Guamanian diet, culture, and lifestyle.[73]

Cycad flour: cycasin and β-N-methylamino-L-alanine (BMAA)

At the district level, we calculated Pearson correlation coefficients for reported mean concentrations (μg/g) of two cycad flour neurotoxins cycasin (methyl-azoxymethanol β-D-glucoside) and BMAA (β-N-methylamino-L-alanine) in cycad flour samples from nine Guam districts.[74] We demonstrated for men and women a highly significant correlation ($P = 0.00002$, $r = 0.98$) between average annual age adjusted incidence rates of motor neuron disease and *cycasin* but not BMMA.[68]

Geochemical elements

Geochemical factors were correlated by using reported mean concentrations (ppm) of selected chemical elements in water and soil samples.[75] We found a statistically significant correlation ($P = 0.0002$, $r = 0.77$ for men, $r = 0.69$ for women) for *high water iron* content in samples from 18 districts, and with *silicon* concentrations in water (for men only).[68] Among soil elements, only *cobalt and nickel* were significant for men and women with motor neuron disease.[68]

Familial occurrence of Guamanian motor neuron disease

Family history was available for 303 Chamorros (187 men, 116 women) who developed motor neuron disease in Guam between 1956 and 1985. Positive family history of documented motor neuron disease was found in 108 (36%), including affected parents in 18, 78 in sibs, and 13 in offspring. Of those with a positive family history, 19 (17·6%) had affected spouses suggesting a high risk of developing motor neuron disease among spouses. There were 160 offspring-producing couples (born before 1921) who had a total of 1335 children of whom 11 (0·85%) were known to have developed motor neuron disease by 1985. There were eight couples where both partners were affected by the disease. They had a total of 69 children of whom two (2·9%) had developed the disease by 1985.

The risk of motor neuron disease in susceptible sibships was about 4·9–15·5% or about seven to 28 times greater than the general population lifetime risk (seven times higher in high rate districts and 28 times higher in low rate districts). These values are lower than expected with Mendelian inheritance, and considering the decline of incidence rates with time, polygenic inheritance alone is also unlikely.

Guamanian motor neuron disease revisited: a unifying hypothesis

Reappraisal of Guamanian ALS data is consistent with a process resulting from genetic susceptibility precipitated by exposure to environmental or exogenous agents during adolescence.

Familial factors

Early in the studies of motor neuron disease on Guam a dominant pattern of inheritance was suggested to explain the familial aggregation.[69] However, it soon became clear that the epidemiology of the disease was inconsistent with Mendelian

179

inheritance.[62 64 70 76] In view of recent progress in the understanding of FALS, it is conceivable that a susceptibility gene could be present among the Chamorro.

We found that the risk of development of motor neuron disease in susceptible sibships was up to 28 times greater than the general population lifetime risk.[68] Unfortunately, to date no genetic studies to define chromosome linkage or known gene products (CuZnSOD deficiency, hexosaminidase A/B deficiency) have been carried out on Guam.

Environmental factors

Regarding the nature of the exogenous agents, the epidemiological evidence favours, with modifications, the two current causal hypotheses—that is, cycad excitotoxins[71] and geochemicals.[72]

Cycas circinalis

There was a highly significant correlation between average annual age adjusted incidence rates of motor neuron disease on Guam and flour content of cycasin—one of the postulated exogenous toxins of *Cycas circinalis*. Most of the experimental work on cycas neurotoxicity was based on chronic BMAA intoxication in monkeys, inducing clinical and pathological features reminiscent of Guamanian ALS-parkinsonism.[71 74 77] Our epidemiological evidence would also provide support for cycas neurotoxicity as an aetiological agent in Guam.[78]

Aluminium and iron

The alternative geochemical hypothesis surmised that low concentrations of calcium and magnesium along with increased aluminum in the soil and water caused Guamanian ALS.[72] This was based on the finding of accumulation of calcium, aluminium, and silicon in neurofibrillary tangle bearing neurons in the brains of patients with Guamanian ALS-parkinsonism-dementia complex.[79] Juvenile primates fed a low calcium diet with or without supplemental aluminium showed neuropathological changes suggestive of those of Guamanian ALS, including neurofibrillary tangles.[80] Intracisternal injections of aluminium chloride in rabbits produced a chronic encephalopathy with impaired axonal transport and inclusions that resembled those of ALS.[81]

We found no correlation of motor neuron disease with calcium, magnesium, or aluminium content in soil and water, as previously reported. None the less, a significant correlation did exist with iron concentrations in water samples.[68]

Iron has been recently implicated in neurodegenerative disorders—mainly Parkinson's disease,[82 83] because of its ability to generate free radicals and to cause oxidative stress.[83] Also, the protein lactotransferrin, which transports iron and other metals, is present in the neuropathological lesions of some degenerative disorders, including most prominently Guamanian ALS-parkinsonism-dementia complex.[84] Lactotransferrin is strongly immunoreactive with Betz cell and with other neurons of the motor cortex affected in ALS,[84] suggesting that increased deposition of iron could be of pathogenetic importance in motor neuron disease by inducing oxidative cytotoxicity.

As in the case of familial ALS associated with deficiency of Cu/Zn superoxide dismustase (SOD1) and in mice transgenic for mutant SOD1, a perturbation in free radical metabolism, perhaps through membrane lipid peroxidation, could be important in motor neuron cell death.[85] In the experimental model in mice, vitamin E, riluzole, and gabapentin influenced the progression of the disease.[86]

Conclusions

Epidemiological evidence on Guam favours the hypothesis of a genetic predisposition to develop motor neuron disease after exposure to environmental excitotoxins or chemicals—in particular, cycas neurotoxins and iron. This view essentially agrees with the postulated pathogenesis of motor neuron disease based on epidemiological studies of an outbreak of motor neuron disease in Sweden.[42] The nature of the genetic susceptibility is unclear but pharmacogenetic polymorphism leading to deficient detoxifying capacity has been suggested.[87] In turn, this might induce release of free radicals, oxidative cytotoxicity, and apoptosis leading to neuronal death.

Geographic isolates of neurodegenerative diseases constitute invaluable "experiments of nature", the lessons of which we are just beginning to discern.

1 Charcot JM. *Lectures on the diseases of the nervous system.* Translated and edited by Sigerson G. Three volumes, second series. London: The New Sydenham Society, 1881.
2 World Federation of Neurology Research Group on Neuromuscular Disorders. Classification of neuromuscular disorders. *J Neurol Sci* 4;**124**(suppl):109–30.
3 World Federation of Neurology Research Group on Neuromuscular Disorders. El Escorial World Federation of Neurology Criteria for the Diagnosis of Amyotrophic Lateral Sclerosis. *J Neurol Sci* 1994;**124**(suppl):96–107.
4 Ray Chaudhuri K, Crump S, al-Sarraj S, Anderson V, Cavanagh J, Leigh PN. The validation of El Escorial criteria for the diagnosis of amyotrophic lateral sclerosis: a clinicopathological study. *J Neurol Sci* 1995;**129** (suppl):11–2.
5 World Health Organisation. *Neurological adaptation of the 10th International Classification of Diseases (ICD-10 NA),* Geneva: WHO, 1994.
6 Armon C. *Motor neuron disease.* In: Gorelick PB, Alter M, eds. *Handbook of neuroepidemiology.* New York: Dekker, 1994:407–54.
7 Chancellor AM, Warlow CP. Adult onset motor neuron disease: worldwide mortality, incidence, and distribution since 1950. *J Neurol Neurosurg Psychiatry* 1992;**55**:1106–15.
8 Rosati G, Granieri E. *Manuale di Neuroepidemiologia Clinica.* Roma: NIS, 1990:295–317.
9 De Pedro-Cuesta J, Litvan I. Epidemiology of motor neuron disease. In: Anderson DW, ed. *Neuroepidemiology: a tribute to Bruce Schoenberg.* Boca Raton: CRC Press, 1991:265–96.
10 Hoffman PM, Brody JA. The reliability of death certificate reporting for amyotrophic lateral sclerosis. *Journal of Chronic Diseases* 1971;**24**:5–8.
11 O'Malley F, Dean G, Elian M. Multiple sclerosis and motor neurone disease: survival and how certified after death. *J Epidemiol Community Health* 1987;**41**:14–7.
12 Chiò A, Magnani C, Oddenino E, Tolardo G, Schiffer D. Accuracy of death certificate diagnosis of amyotrophic lateral sclerosis. *J Epidemiol Community Health* 1992;**46**:517–8.
13 Chancellor AM, Swingler RJ, Fraser H, Clarke JA, Warlow CP. Utility of Scottish morbidity and mortality data for epidemiological studies of motor neuron disease. *J Epidemiol Community Health* 1993;**47**:116–20.
14 Neilson S, Gunnarsson L-G, Robinson I. Rising mortality from motor neuron disease in Sweden 1961–1990: the relative role of increased population life expectancy and environmental factors. *Acta Neurol Scand* 1994;**90**:150–9.
15 Elian M, Dean G. The changing mortality from motor neuron disease and multiple sclerosis in England and Wales and the Republic of Ireland. *Neuroepidemiology* 1991;**11**:236–43.
16 Leone M, Chandra V, Schoenberg BS. Motor neuron disease in the United States, 1971 and 1973–1978. *Neurology* 1987;**37**:1339–43.
17 Neilson S, Robinson I, Hunter M. Longitudinal Gompertzian analysis of ALS mortality in England and Wales, 1963–1989: estimates of susceptibility in the general population. *Mech Ageing Dev* 1992;**64**:201–16.
18 Jokelainen M. The epidemiology of amyotrophic lateral sclerosis in Finland. *J Neurol Sci* 1976;**29**:55–63.
19 Neilson S, Robinson I, Alperovitch A. Rising amyotrophic lateral sclerosis mortality in France, 1968–1990: increased life expectancy and inter-disease competition as an explanation. *J Neurol* 1994;**241**:448–55.
20 Chiò A, Magnani C, Schiffer D. Amyotrophic lateral sclerosis in Italy, 1958 to 1987: a cross-sectional and cohort study. *Neurology* 1993;**43**:927–30.
21 Neilson S, Robinson I, Nymoen EH. Longitudinal analysis of amyotrophic lateral sclerosis mortality in Norway, 1966–1989: evidence for a susceptible subpopulation. *J Neurol Sci* 1994;**122**:148–54.

182

22 Neilson S, Robinson I, Kondo K. A new analysis of mortality from motor neuron disease in Japan, 1950–1990: rise and fall in the postwar years. *J Neurol Sci* 1993;**117**:46–53.

23 Lilienfeld DE, Chan E, Ehland J, *et al*. Rising mortality from motor neuron disease in the USA, 1962–1984. *Lancet* 1988;**i**:710–3.

24 Riggs JE. Longitudinal Gompertzian analysis of amyotrophic lateral sclerosis mortality in the USA, 1977–1986: evidence for an inherently susceptible population subset. *Mech Ageing Dev* 1990;**55**:207–20.

25 Román GC, Zhang Z-X, Ellenberg JH. The neuroepidemiology of Parkinson's disease. In: Ellenberg JH, Koller WC, Langston JW, eds. *Etiology of Parkinson's disease*. New York: Dekker, 1995:203–43.

26 Chiò A, Meineri P, Tribolo A, Schiffer D. Risk factors in motor neuron disease: a case-control study. *Neuroepidemiology* 1991;**10**:174–84.

27 Granieri E, Rosati G, Paolino E, Tola R, Aiello I, Granieri S. The risk of amyotrophic lateral sclerosis among laborers in Sardinia, Italy: a case-control study [abstract]. *J Neurol* 1985;**232**(suppl):15.30.

28 Holloway S, Emery AEH. The epidemiology of motor neuron disease in Scotland. *Muscle Nerve* 1982;**5**:131–3.

29 Giagheddu M, Puggioni G, Masala C, *et al*. Epidemiologic study of amyotrophic lateral sclerosis in Sardinia, Italy. *Acta Neurol Scand* 1983;**68**:394–404.

30 Bharucha NE, Schoenberg BS, Raven RH, Pickle LW, Byar DP, Mason TJ. Geographic distribution of motor neuron disease and correlation with possible etiologic factors. *Neurology* 1983;**33**:911–5.

31 Granieri E, Carreras M, Tola R, Paolino E, Troill G, Eleofra R, Serra G. Motor neuron disease in the Province of Ferrara, Italy, 1964–1982. *Neurology* 1988;**38**:1604–8.

32 Angelini C, Armani M, Bresolin N. Incidence and risk factors of motor neuron disease in the Venice and Padua districts of Italy, 1972–1979. *Neuroepidemiology* 1983;**2**:236–40.

33 Hochberg FH, Bryan JA, Whelan MA. Clustering of amyotrophic lateral sclerosis. *Lancet* 1974;**i**:34.

34 Melmed C, Krieger C. A cluster of amyotrophic lateral sclerosis. *Arch Neurol* 1982;**39**:595–6.

35 Sanders M. Clustering of amyotrophic lateral sclerosis. *JAMA* 1980;**244**:435.

36 Hyser CL, Kissel JT, Mendell JR. Three cases of amyotrophic lateral sclerosis in a common occupational environment. *J Neurol* 1987;**234**:443–4.

37 Proctor SP, Feldman RG, Wolf PA, Brent B, Wartenberg D. A perceived cluster of amyotrophic lateral sclerosis in a Massachusetts community. *Neuroepidemiology* 1992;**1**:277–81.

38 Armon C, Daube JR, O'Brien PC, Kurland LT, Mulder DW. When is an apparent excess of neurologic cases epidemiologically significant? *Neurology* 1991;**41**:1713–8.

39 Gunnarsson L-G, Lindberg G, Söderfeldt B, Axelson O. The mortality of motor neuron disease in Sweden 1961–85. *Arch Neurol* 1990;**47**:42–6.

40 Gunnarsson L-G, Lygner P-E, Veiga-Cabo J, De-Pedro-Cuesta J. An epidemic-like cluster of motor neuron disease in a Swedish county during the period 1973–1984. *Neuroepidemiology* 1995;.

41 Gunnarsson L-G, Bodin G, Söderfeldt B, Axelson O. A case-control study of motor neuron disease: its relation to heritability, and occupational exposures, particularly to solvents. *Br J Ind Med* 1992;**49**:791–8.

42 Gunnarsson L-G. Motor neuron disease and exposure to chemicals—aetiological suggestions from a case-control study. *J Neurol Sci* 1994;**124**(suppl):62–3.

43 Kurtzke JF. Risk factors in amyotrophic lateral sclerosis. *Adv Neurol* 1991;**56**:245–70.

44 Kurland LT, Radhakrishnan K, Smith GE, Armon G, Nemetz PN. Mechanical trauma as a risk factor in classic amyotrophic lateral sclerosis: lack of epidemiologic evidence. *J Neurol Sci* 1992;**113**:133–43.

45 Appel SH, Smith RG, Engelhardt JI, Stefani E. Evidence for autoimmunity in amyotrophic lateral sclerosis. *J Neurol Sci* 1994;**124**(suppl):14–9.

46 Rowland LP. Amyotrophic lateral sclerosis with paraproteins and auto-antibodies. *Adv Neurol* 1995;**68**:93–105.

47 Swingler RJ, Fraser H, Harlow CP. Motor neuron disease and polio in Scotland. *J Neurol Neurosurg Psychiatry* 1992;**55**:1116–20.

48 Okumura H, Kurland LT, Waring SC. Amyotrophic lateral sclerosis and polio: is there an association? *Ann NY Acad Sci* 1995;**753**:245–56.

49 Román GC, Vernant J-C, Osame M. HTLV-I-associated motor neuron disease. *Handbook Clin Neurol* 1991;**59**:447–57.

50 Ferrante P, Westarp ME, Mancuso R, *et al.* HTLV tax-rex DNA and antibodies in idiopathic amyotrophic lateral sclerosis. *J Neurol Sci* 1995;**129**(suppl):140–4.

51 Westarp ME, Ferrante P, Perron H, Bartmann P, Kornhuber HH. Sporadic ALS/MND: a global neurodegeneration with retroviral involvement. *J Neurol Sci* 1995;**129**(suppl):145–7.

52 Wiedau-Pazos M, Goto JJ, Rabizadeh S, *et al.* Altered reactivity of superoxide dismutase in familial amyotrophic lateral sclerosis. *Science* 1996;**271**:515–8.

53 Plaitikis A, Caroscio JT. Abnormal glutamate metabolism in amyotrophic lateral sclerosis. *Ann Neurol* 1987;**22**:575–9.

54 Plaitikis A, Mandeli J, Fesdjian C, Sivak MA. Dysregulation of glutamate metabolism in ALS: correlation with gender and disease type. *Neurology* 1991;**41**:392–3.

55 Rothstein JD, Tsai G, Kuncl RW, *et al.* Abnormal excitatory amino acid metabolism in amyotrophic lateral sclerosis. *Ann Neurol* 1990;**28**:18–25.

56 Rothstein JD, Martin LJ, Kuncl RW. Decreased glutamate transport by the brain and spinal cord in amyotrophic lateral sclerosis. *N Engl J Med* 1992;**326**:1464–8.

57 Shaw PJ. Excitotoxicity and motor neurone disease: a review of the evidence. *J Neurol Sci* 1994;**24**(suppl):6–13.

58 Bensimon G, Lacomblez L, Meininger V, ALS/Riluzole Study Group. A controlled trial of riluzole in amyotrophic lateral sclerosis. *N Engl J Med* 1994;**330**:585–91.

59 Gourie-Devi M, ed. *Motor neuron disease: global clinical patterns and international research*. New Delhi: Oxford and IBH Publishing Co, 1988.

60 Hentati A, Bejaoui K, Pericak-Vance MA, *et al.* Linkage of recessive familial amyotrophic lateral sclerosis to chromosome 2q33-q35. *ACI Nature Genetics* 1994;**7**:425–8.

61 Kurland LT, Mulder DW. Epidemiologic investigations of amyotrophic lateral sclerosis. I. Preliminary report on geographic distribution, with special reference to the Mariana Islands, including clinical and pathologic observations. *Neurology* 1954;**4**:355–78.

62 Reed DM, Brody JA. Amyotrophic lateral sclerosis and parkinsonism-dementia on Guam, 1945–1972. I: Descriptive epidemiology. *Am J Epidemiol* 1975;**101**:287–301.

63 Garruto RM, Yanagihara R, Gajdusek DC. Disappearance of high-incidence amyotrophic lateral sclerosis and parkinsonism-dementia on Guam. *Neurology* 1985;**35**:193–8.

64 Reed D, Labarthe D, Chen KM, Stallones R. A cohort study of amyotrophic lateral sclerosis and parkinsonism-dementia on Guam and Rota. *Am J Epidemiol* 1987;**125**:92–100.

65 Araki S, Iwasashi Y, Kuroiwa Y. Epidemiological study of amyotrophic lateral sclerosis and allied disorders in the Kii Peninsula (Japan). *J Neurol Sci* 1967;**4**:279–82.

66 Gajdusek DC, Salazar AM. Amyotrophic lateral sclerosis and parkinsonian syndromes in high incidence among the Auyu and Jakai people of West New Guinea. *Neurology* 1982;**32**:107–26.

67 Zhang ZX, Anderson DW, Mantel N, Román GC. Motor neuron disease on Guam. Temporal occurrence, 1941–85. *Acta Neurol Scand* 1995;**92**:299–307.

68 Zhang ZX, Anderson DW, Mantel N, Román GC. Motor neuron disease on Guam: geographic and familial occurrence, 1956–85. *Acta Neurol Scand* 1996;**94**:51–9.

69 Kurland LT, Mulder DW. Epidemiologic investigations of amyotrophic lateral sclerosis. II. Familial aggregations indicative of dominant inheritance, part 1. *Neurology* 1955;**5**:182–96.

70 Reed DM, Torres JM, Brody JA. Amyotrophic lateral sclerosis and parkinsonism-dementia on Guam, 1945–1972. II: Familial and genetic studies. *Am J Epidemiol* 1975;**101**:302–10.

71 Spencer PS, Nunn PB, Hugon J, et al. Guam amyotrophic lateral sclerosis-Parkinsonism-dementia linked to a plant excitant neurotoxin. *Science* 1987;**237**:517–22.

72 Garruto RM. Neurotoxicity of trace and essential elements: factors provoking the high incidence of motor neuron disease, Parkinsonism and dementia in the Western Pacific. In: Gouri-Devi M, ed: *Motor neurone disease: global clinical patterns and international research.* New Delhi: Oxford and IBH Publishing Co, 1987:73–82.

73 Steele JC, Guzman T. Observations about amyotrophic lateral sclerosis and the Parkinsonism-dementia complex of Guam with regard to epidemiology and etiology. *Can J Neurol Sci* 1987;**14**(suppl):358–62.

74 Kisby GE, Ellison M, Spencer PS. Content of the neurotoxins cycasin (methylazoxymethanol β-D-glucoside) and BMAA (β-N-methylamino-L-alanine) in cycad flour prepared by Guam Chamorros. *Neurology* 1992;**42**:1336–40.

75 Garruto RM, Yanagihara R, Gajdusek DC, Arion DM. Concentrations of heavy metals and essential minerals in garden soil and drinking water in the western Pacific. In: Chen KM, Chase Y, eds. *Amyotrophic lateral sclerosis in Asia and Oceania.* Taiwan, Republic of China: National Taiwan University, 1984:265–330.

76 Kurland LT, Molgaard CA. Guamanian ALS: hereditary or acquired? In: Rowland LP, ed. *Human motor neuron diseases.* New York: Raven Press, 1982:165–71.

77 Kisby GE, Ross SM, Spencer PS, et al. Cycasin and BMAA: Candidate neurotoxins for western Pacific amyotrophic lateral sclerosis/parkinsonism-dementia complex. *Neurodegeneration* 1992;**1**:73–82.

78 Spencer PS, Kisby GE, Ross SM, Roy DN, Hugon J, Ludolph AC, Nunn PB. Guam ALS-PDC: possible causes. *Science* 1993;**262**:825–6.

79 Perl DP, Gajdusek DC, Garruto RM, Yanagihara RT, Gibbs CJ. Intraneuronal aluminum accumulation in amyotrophic lateral sclerosis and Parkinsonism-dementia of Guam. *Science* 1982;**217**:1053–5.

80 Garruto RM, Shankar SK, Yanagihara R, Salazar AM, Amyx HL, Gajdusek DC. Low calcium, high aluminum diet-induced motor neuron pathology in cynomolgus monkeys. *Acta Neuropathol* 1989;**78**:210–9.

81 Strong MJ, Garruto RM. Chronic aluminum-induced motor neuron degeneration: clinical, neuropathological and molecular biological aspects. *Can J Neurol Sci* 1991;**18**:431.

82 Jellinger K, Kienzl E. Iron deposits in brain disorders. In: Riederer P, Youdim MBH, eds. *Iron in central nervous system disorders.* New York: Springer Verlag, 1993:19–36.

83 Koeppen AH, ed. Normal and pathological brain iron. *J Neurol Sci* 1995;**134**(suppl):1–114.

84 Levuegle B, Spik G, Perl DP, Bouras C, Fillit HM, Hof PR. The iron-binding protein lactotransferrin is present in pathological lesions in a variety of neurodegenerative disorders: a comparative immunohistochemical analysis. *Brain Res* 1994;**650**:20–31.

85 Brown RH. Superoxide dismutase and familial amyotrophic lateral sclerosis: new insights into mechanisms and treatments. *Ann Neurol* 1996;**39**:145–6.

86 Gurney ME, Cutting FB, Zhai P, Doble A, Taylor CP, Andrus PK, Hall ED. Benefit of vitamin E, riluzole and gabapentin in a transgenic model of familial amyotrophic lateral sclerosis. *Ann Neurol* 1996;**39**:147–57.

87 Heafield MT, Fearn S, Stevenson GB, Waring RH, Williams AC, Sturman SG. Plasma cysteine and sulphate levels in patients with motor neurone, Parkinson's and Alzheimer's disease. *Neurosci Lett* 1990;**110**:216–20.

9 Multiple sclerosi

ALASTAIR COMPSTON, NEIL ROBER

- Epidemiological investigation of multiple scler has been dominated by prevalence surveys.
- There are large variations in prevalence between different parts of the world.
- The results of migrant studies show that environmental factors are likely to influence risk of multiple sclerosis.
- Pedigree analysis and molecular studies also show a genetic contribution to susceptibility.
- The incomplete concordance rate among monozygotic twins indicates a modifying effect of the environment on genetic susceptibility.

Epidemiological studies of multiple sclerosis have been performed on almost an industrial scale over the past 90 years. Morbidity statistics have been used to generate aetiological hypotheses, to assess local needs for the provision of services and the allocation of resources, and to define the natural history of the disease. Methodological factors have limited the extent to which the many surveys have yielded definitive conclusions in any one of these contexts. Most vulnerable have been the comparisons of prevalence between regions and the serial studies of single places.

In planning an epidemiological study in multiple sclerosis, the usual practice is to retrieve cases from lists of those already known to be affected. Because in most parts of the world the diagnosis is coordinated through hospital clinics, scrutiny of departmental and office notes provides the best source of information. In some situations, a case can be made for retrospectively adjusting statistics to include those people who would have featured in a population based survey if their whereabouts or clinical status had been known at the time (onset adjusted prevalence[1]); their exclusion can then be regarded as an error of administration, recognition, disease expression, or any one of the quirks which makes one person seek medical advice in advance of another. Rigid application of criteria for inclusion, and the decision to omit suspected cases, will vary depending on the purposes of the study. For surveys examining biological features, the error should be

.rds inclusion of those who *probably* have the disease process
.ven if this is not yet clinically declared. In other contexts, it is
essential to restrict the register to those who *definitely* have the
disease.

Cases of different racial origin should not be grouped because
they may differ for important characteristics. Sociohistorical
factors are known to create significant differences in risk status
even across quite small regions; conversely, some questions
relating to the epidemiology of multiple sclerosis, which involve
cohort studies, can only be answered by comparing specifically
different locations. It makes little sense to plan a study requiring
the recruitment of significant numbers of patients with a rare
manifestation of multiple sclerosis, such as twinning or familial
disease, in a community which has a low overall prevalence of the
disease. Similarly, a ubiquitous but biologically important feature
may not differ significantly between groups in places where
multiple sclerosis is relatively common. It follows that there are
usually better opportunites for identifying risk factors which make
a significant contribution to the disease but are frequent in the at
risk population by working in areas of low prevalence; conversely,
risk factors for multiple sclerosis which are not overrepresented in
the normal population will be identified more easily in high
prevalence regions.

The extent to which complete ascertainment is achieved
depends much on the structure, size, and distribution of the
denominator, and whether the population has previously been
surveyed. The few patients with multiple sclerosis in a medium to
low prevalence island community with a demographically stable
population of around 20 000 and a normal age structure, can
easily be ascertained but when surveying the disease in one at risk
group living within a large metropolitan but ethnically mixed
community, it may prove impossible to ascertain with confidence
either the numerator or denominator, especially if recent
population censuses are not available. Improved provision of
facilities for the disabled inflates both prevalence and mortality;
and the arrival of an investigator with a special interest in the
disease abruptly increases morbidity estimates although these will
plateau once ascertainment is saturated. Underestimating the
absolute number of cases may not affect the definition of
geographical gradients in the distribution of multiple sclerosis but
it does matter in serial studies of a single region where a rise in
prevalence resulting from reduced mortality and altered

188

diagnostic criteria has to be distinguished from a real increase in incidence. It follows that investigator vigilance is a major confounding factor in comparative epidemiology.

Distribution of multiple sclerosis

By the beginning of the 20th century, multiple sclerosis—a disease that merited individual case reports 25 years previously—had become one of the commonest reasons for admission to a neurological ward. The period 1900 to 1950 saw a gradual evolution of methods required for accurate definition of population based statistics; over the past four decades, surveys from most parts of the world have established the *big picture* on the geography of the disease and have allowed speculation on the reasons for its characteristic distribution.

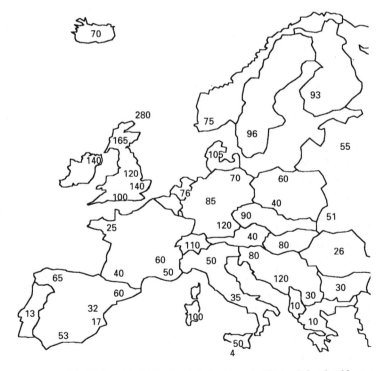

Figure 9.1   Distribution of multiple sclerosis in Scandinavia (Finland, Sweden, Norway, Denmark, and Iceland), central Europe (Holland, Switzerland, Austria, Germany, Hungary, Slovakia, Poland), France, Spain and Portugal, Italy, Malta, Greece, Albania, Croatia, Romania, and Bulgaria; figures are prevalence/10⁵ of the population.

189

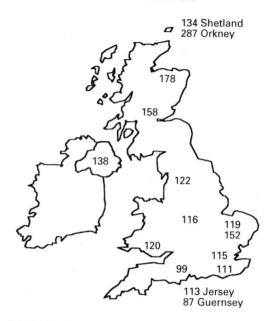

Figure 9.2   Distribution of multiple sclerosis in the United Kingdom; figures are prevalence/10⁵ of the population.

Twenty years ago John Kurtzke, who has worked hardest to make sense of the epidemiological facts relating to multiple sclerosis, collated the published surveys of prevalence and suggested that the distribution could broadly be classified into bands of low, medium, and high prevalence.[2-4] High risk (>30/10⁵) was found throughout northern Europe, the northern United States, Canada, southern Australia, and New Zealand; medium risk (5–30/10⁵) was found in southern Europe, the southern United States and northern Australia; and low risk (<5/10⁵) areas included Asia, South America, and many uncharted regions. Systematic updating of these figures shows that the absolute number of cases identified in different parts of the world has risen steadily since the 1950s.[5-7] Rather than catalogue all the surveys (now running to many hundreds) or describe the laborious evolution of the ideas on causation which flow from them, figs 9.1–9.4 depict surveys for the regional prevalences of multiple sclerosis in 1997 in Europe, the United Kingdom, North America and Canada, and Australasia: there is a relative paucity of information on incidence; individual sources of information are not cited; nor are 95% confidence intervals (95% CIs) shown as

190

these are not always provided in the original publications and some of the figures are a best guess. The figures for the United Kingdom in fig 9.1 are regional approximations for those given in fig 9.2. What emerges from the more recent surveys is that many of the putative claims for latitudinal gradients were overstated but it remains the case that the disease does show variations in its distribution over quite small distances which may be informative with respect to ideas on the aetiology.

Multiple sclerosis is evidently a common disorder of young adults in northern Europe, continental North America (see figure 9.3) and Australasia (see figure 9.4) but not in the Orient, the Arabian peninsula, Africa, continental South America, and India. Nevertheless, in northern Europe, prevalence (and incidence) are higher in southern Scandinavia, northern Germany, the United Kingdom and parts of Italy, than in northern Scandinavia, France, Spain, and the eastern Mediterranean countries. Within the United Kingdom, the disease is more prevalent in north east Scotland, and the Orkney and Shetland islands than in other parts of England, Wales, and Ireland.[8] In Italy, pronounced differences in prevalence exist between regions and islands that are geographically close but differ in their genetic and cultural histories.[9] In north America, there is a diagonal gradient in frequency with the highest rates in the midwest and the lowest in the Missisippi delta.[10] The comprehensive survey from Australia, in which four regions were surveyed simultaneously using comparable methods and working to a common prevalence date also shows a latitudinal gradient for the white Australian population with higher rates in the south than in the north.[11]

Multiple sclerosis in migrants

Populations are neither geographically nor socially stable and there have been many migrations involving relatively large numbers of people which seem to have influenced the distribution of multiple sclerosis. Whereas studies of stable indigenous populations illustrate differences in genetic susceptibility, the effect of migration has been to define multiple sclerosis as an acquired exogenous disorder.

Attention was first paid to comparisons of the frequency of multiple sclerosis between racial groups in a single geographical setting in South Africa during the 1950s. Dean showed that age

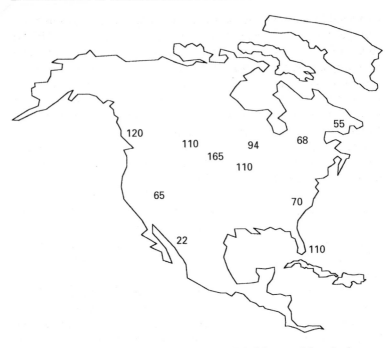

Figure 9.3   Distribution of multiple sclerosis in the United States and Canada; figures are prevalence/10^5 of the population.

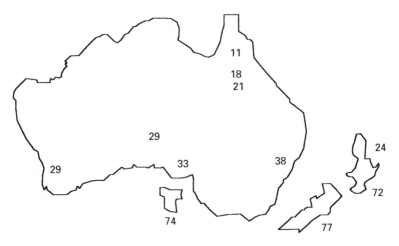

Figure 9.4   Distribution of multiple sclerosis in Australia and New Zealand; figures are prevalence/10^5 of the population.

corrected frequency of the disease was highest in immigrants from Europe, low in Afrikaaners, and intermediate in South African English for both prevalence and incidence[12]; the absolute absence of multiple sclerosis in African black people was confirmed but a slightly higher rate was seen in the Cape Coloured population, which has mixed African and European ancestry. Within the English speaking white population, those moving from northern Europe to southern Africa as adults took with them the high frequency of the country of origin, whereas those migrating younger than 15 years showed the lower rates characteristic of native born inhabitants of southern Africa.

No less influential has been the study of United Kingdom born children of immigrants from the Indian subcontinent, Africa, and the West Indies,[13 14] which showed that the prevalence of multiple sclerosis in the United Kingdom born children of West Indian, African, and Asian immigrants approximates to that seen in similar age groups among the white population. Although methodological difficulties arise in this study of an ethnic minority living in a large metropolis, there are several reasons for suspecting that the number of patients with multiple sclerosis, born in the United Kingdom of parents who were migrants from the West Indies, Africa, or Asia, has actually been underascertained. However, the danger of extrapolating from studies involving a small numerator living in an unusual environment is well illustrated by the study of multiple sclerosis among immigrants from Vietnam to Paris, France.[15] Three cases were identified among a cohort of around 3400 persons born of Vietnamese mothers who came to France under the age of 20 years. The fact that the cumulative 18 year risk of multiple sclerosis, by 1975, was $89/10^5$ (95% CI 18–260), with an age specific prevalence of $169/10^5$ (95% CI 94–135) in the third decade actually tells us nothing about the shift in risk of the disease consequent on movement of people from southern Asia to northern France as, apart from the wide confidence intervals, having a French born father was a requirement for immigration; genetic admixture therefore introduced an essential bias into this study.

Another classic series of epidemiological studies compared the frequency of multiple sclerosis among Japanese in Hawaii, the west coast of North America, and Japan. In Hawaii, the prevalence among Japanese was $7/10^5$ compared with $34/10^5$ in white immigrants to Hawaii[16-18]; these rates were virtually identical for Japanese and white people living in California[19] and can be compared with the expected rate of 2/10[5] for native Japanese.[20] Here, the evidence favours a strong protective effect for the Japanese irrespective of environment.

The other location where migration has occurred on a sufficient scale to show important age related differences in prevalence of multiple sclerosis is Israel. The original study in immigrants reported a difference in prevalence between migrants from northern Europe (Ashkenazi Jews) and from Asia and Africa (Sephardic Jews).[21 22] The higher frequency in Ashkenazi than Sephardic Jews also showed an age at migration effect, in that there were very few Ashkenazis in the cohort arriving in Israel before adolescence. Although crude rates retained the difference seen in the parental groups, prevalence in the Israeli born children of Ashkenazi and Sephardic Jews was the same after age adjustment to the population of the United States. These important studies have recently been updated[23]; depending on place of paternal birth, prevalence (age adjusted to the Israeli population of 1960) was estimated at 32 (fathers born in Israel), 38 (fathers born in Europe or North America), and 29 (fathers born in Africa or Asia) compared with 14/10[5] in immigrants. Higher rates were found in Jerusalem (61, 68, and 51/10[5] for Israelis with Israeli, European/American, and African/Asian fathers respectively) than in other parts of the country. The implication is that, at least for Ashkenazi and Sephardic Jews, racially determined differences in risk for multiple sclerosis are modified by environment.

Movements within one continent or country are also informative for the assessment of risk depending on time spent in regions of differing prevalence. A study of United States citizens showed that mortality for southern born patients dying in the north was 0·68/10[5]/year compared with 0·46/10[5]/year for those remaining in the south. The mortality ratio for United States army veterans born in the high frequency northern states and entering military service from the middle zone dropped from 1·48 to 1·27, and to 0·74 for those entering from the southern states. Those born in the medium risk zone showed a ratio increase in frequency of multiple sclerosis to 1·4 if entering military service from the north and a reduced ratio of 0·73 if entering from the south.[24]

All of these studies proved enormously influential in shaping ideas on the contribution of environmental factors to the aetiology of multiple sclerosis. Having established from the migration studies and analyses of epidemics that environmental factors

194

probably do alter the risks of developing multiple sclerosis, and may *override* racial susceptibility, it became important to establish at what age these influences occur. Clearly, the critical period is before clinical onset and the studies from South Africa and the United States veterans' survey suggest that, in all probability, the disease process is established in childhood but few would be confident about confining risk to a particular calender age.

As part of a national survey of multiple sclerosis in France, 246 persons were identified who had migrated from north Africa in the first quinquennium of the 1960s after the Algerian war for independence, among 8000 cases ascertained overall in France.[25] Excluding the 27 patients who had multiple sclerosis before, or at the time of migration, 86% of these 246 probands were European in origin and the remainder Arab or Berber. There was no apparent age or sex adjusted difference in frequency or mean age at onset between these and native French cases and this has been interpreted as indicating that the provocative exogenous factors are ubiquitous and that multiple sclerosis is acquired by the same age in each group. As far as this study is concerned, Kurtzke considers that matching by age has introduced a confounding factor as this will have restricted individual subjects to those with the same age at onset; he prefers the interpretation that in this cohort there is a fixed interval between migration and clinical onset, regardless of age, and takes the study to provide evidence for susceptibility extending to people in the mid-40s.[7] However, a range of more than 30 years could be considered not to provide much insight into the critical age of exposure to the putative agent which causes multiple sclerosis.

Epidemics of multiple sclerosis

Those who espouse the environmental doctrine of multiple sclerosis are naturally enthusiastic about epidemics of the disease. The arguments put forward by Kurtzke[7] for point source epidemics, especially that proposed for the Faroe Islands, have not been universally accepted and others take the view that these are epidemics of recognition reflecting the arrival of specialist medical services in island communities rather than a genuine change in incidence arising from the introduction of transmissible aetiological factors into virgin populations.

195

In the first survey of Iceland, 168 cases of multiple sclerosis were identified with onset between 1900 and 1975.[26] Annual incidence rates seemed to rise around 1922; they then stabilised until a further increase occurred in 1945, heralding a steady decline from the mid-1950s. Each quinquennial rate for incidence from 1900 was lower than between 1945 and 1954, during which age at onset was also younger than before or after this period. This led to the conclusion that there had been a postwar epidemic of multiple sclerosis in Iceland[26 27] but opinions differ both with respect to the facts and their interpretation. John Benedikz, an Icelandic neurologist who has taken a particular interest in the epidemiology of multiple sclerosis, favours the view that any change in frequency of multiple sclerosis in Iceland during the 20th century should be attributed to improved recognition and diagnostic procedures rather than increased incidence.[1 28] In support of this interpretation, Benedikz et al have reviewed 323 patients with onset of symptoms attributed to multiple sclerosis after 1 January 1900 of whom 252 were still living in December 1989.[29] Incidence rates were $<1/10^5$/year up until the 1930s but then increased to $2·5/10^5$/year, coinciding with the arrival of two neurologists. With waning enthusiasm, so the analysis goes, there was then a lull between 1945 and 1955, when incidence increased to $3·3/10^5$/year after the first systematic survey of the disease. With nine neurologists in practice from 1975, there was a further increase to a peak incidence of $4·1/10^5$/year, which is being maintained. Benedicz et al argue that case ascertainment in the era before 1950 was far from adequate as shown by the long interval at that time between onset and diagnosis, with a paucity of milder registered cases, and comparisons of disability in the affected cohorts showing an overloading of those with severe multiple sclerosis before 1950. The abrupt reduction in interval between onset and diagnosis after 1940 is seen as further evidence for the impact of neurological expertise on early diagnosis and improved case ascertainment.

The original findings on multiple sclerosis in the Faroe islands[30 31] showed fewer cases than expected from comparisons with neighbouring Orkney and Shetland. Kurtzke[7] searched many places in his attempt to trace cases back to before the second world war but in neither the initial survey[31] nor later assessments[32-35] was any patient identified with an estimated date of onset earlier than 1943. There were then 16 cases with onset between 1943 and 1949, a further 16 developing clinical manifestations between 1950 and 1973 and, by 1986, 41 patients had been ascertained of whom nine had lived abroad for three or more years and so were not considered directly to have been part of the epidemic. Kurtzke concludes that the critical factor determining the Faroes experience of multiple sclerosis was occupation by British troops between 1940 and 1945, the development of multiple sclerosis showing both a temporal and spatial relation in that villages where people lived who contributed to each of the incidence peaks were also those where troops were billeted. But some are not convinced by this analysis[36][37] despite robust counter claims from the main protagonists with respect to specific criticisms concerning validity of the diagnoses, exclusions, case ascertainment, definition of epidemics, and the putative role of the British occupation in the genesis of this cluster.[7][35]

In the Orkney and Shetland Islands, the incidence and prevalence of multiple sclerosis were at one time higher, almost by an order of magnitude, than in other regions. Estimates of prevalence carried out on four occasions between 1954 and 1974 showed a steady rise in frequency from $111/10^5$ in 1954 to $309/10^5$ in 1974 for Orkney, and from $134/10^5$ to $184/10^5$ in Shetland over the same period.[8][38] Comparison of incidence and mortality confirms the impression that there has been no significant alteration in statistics for the disease other than those attributable to changes in classification and ascertainment. Over the period of these studies, systematic depopulation in Orkney and Shetland left an older population less at risk of multiple sclerosis and, as elsewhere, the rise in prevalence can best be attributed to increased survival (from 26 to 40 years in Orkney and from 24–34 years in Shetland between 1954 and 1974) and improved case recognition. The question of serial change in incidence for multiple sclerosis in Orkney has since been revisited; although there had been a steady reduction from 1964, prevalence figures for 1994 were $287/10^5$ (probable and definite cases) and $134/10^5$ for Orkney and Shetland respectively (S Cook, personal communication). These statistics show that although there has been significantly less multiple sclerosis in Shetland since 1965, this is no longer true for Orkney.

An epidemic has been claimed for Key West, a tropical island off the west coast of Florida where 37 patients with peak onset in and around 1977–9 were identified in 1984 (prevalence $140/10^5$)—an increase that could not be attributed to alterations in clinical vigilance or differential migration of symptomatic persons to a more favourable climate.[39]

Factors which predict the clinical course

Apart from surveys which have assessed highly selected populations of patients, multiple sclerosis is almost always found to be more common in females than in males. The reported figures vary but a sex ratio of two females:one male is usual, irrespective of ethnicity[40 41]; in children, the excess of females is even more pronounced[42] whereas multiple sclerosis presenting in or beyond the fifth decade more commonly affects males.[40 41]

At diagnosis, many patients with multiple sclerosis want information on the prognosis. So-called *benign* multiple sclerosis is characterised by young age at onset, usually occurring in females with infrequent sensory episodes which recover fully; conversely, the prognosis is more predictably gloomy in males with older age of onset and a progressive course involving motor systems. The influence of attack rate early in the disease on outcome has been somewhat less clear. Whereas all neurologists will be familiar with patients in whom a brisk start to the disease with several nasty attacks settled down into a much more favourable middle and long term course than had at first seemed probable, the large population based studies have shown that attack rate in the early years is of some prognostic value.[40 41 43]

Trauma as a trigger of disease activity in multiple sclerosis has been much considered, and still features in the law courts, where plaintiffs may claim that an accident has provoked the first appearance of multiple sclerosis or altered the course of pre-existing manifestations. Sibley *et al*[44] prospectively studied disease activity by questionnaire and physical examination for eight years. Taking either the three or six month period after each event as *at risk*, only electrical trauma showed an association with new episodes; all other noted forms of trauma were negatively correlated both with clinical exacerbations and disease progression. Siva *et al*,[45] using the Mayo Clinic cohort, also conclude that disease exacerbations are no more frequent in the six months after limb fracture than at other times.

The situation with respect to the risk from anaesthesia is unsatisfactory in that no epidemiologically based studies have been performed and the evidence is entirely anecdotal; some neurologists advise patients to avoid elective interventions while remaining sensible about treatments or procedures which justify the small risk of increasing disease activity—if it actually exists.[46 47]

Several authors have shown prospectively that new episodes of demyelination increase after (presumed) viral exposure but no single agent has been implicated[48 49]; 9% of presumed infections are followed by relapse and 27% of new episodes are related to infection; the relative risk for relapse in the four week period after upper respiratory (especially adenovirus) or gastrointestinal infections is 1·3.

Anecdotal evidence on whether pregnancy affects the immediate or long term course of multiple sclerosis has now been supplemented by prospective surveys which indicate that the onset of multiple sclerosis does not cluster around pregnancy, and that having children does not alter the long term course of the disease but there is an increase in relapse rate during the puerperium. However, a major confounder in the detailed interpretation of these studies is the decision by women with severe disability not to embark on pregnancy and the corresponding preparedness of those with mild disease to start or extend their families. The prospective studies indicate a roughly threefold higher risk in the three to six months after term than during pregnancy,[50 51] and suggest that the attacks may be more severe.[52] There is less agreement on whether or not the relapse rate is maintained or falls during the pregnancy itself, as was suggested in several of the retrospective surveys.[53-55] In the most comprehensive epidemiological analysis of issues relating to multiple sclerosis and pregnancy, Runmarker and Andersen[56] studied an inception cohort in Goteborg, Sweden and disposed of the hypothesis that the onset of multiple sclerosis is influenced by pregnancy; there was a conspicuous absence of onset bouts during pregnancy compared with non-pregnant epochs including the puerperal eight months. Fecundity was reduced in women with multiple sclerosis, presumably by choice, especially in the context of significant disability and this is the probable explanation for the conclusion that pregnancy after onset is associated with a lower risk of progression.

Familial multiple sclerosis

Multiple sclerosis has a familial recurrence rate of about 15% and it is usually assumed that this is due to coinheritance of susceptibility factors, but the alternative hypothesis is that this results from common exposure to environmental factors in childhood. The most comprehensive study of recurrence (from Canada) takes as its baseline a lifetime risk of 0·2% for the entire population, and shows an increase to 3% in other first degree relatives (relative risk 20) and 1% in second degree relatives (relative risk 5·5).[57]

Comparable studies from the United Kingdom confirm that the highest age adjusted recurrence rate is for sisters (4·4%) and brothers (3·2%), compared with parents (2·1%) and offspring (1·8%). Overall, the reduction in risk changes from 2·8% (relative risk 9·2) in first degree relatives to 1·0% (relative risk 3·4) and 0·9% (relative risk 2·9) in second and third degree relatives, respectively, compared with a background age adjusted risk in this population of 0·3%.[58] In Flanders, the recurrence risks are 10-fold to 12-fold for first degree and threefold for second degree relatives.[59]

With some variations in methodology, three recent studies approximate to a population based series of multiple sclerosis in twins.[60-63] Two show remarkable consistency in demonstrating a higher clinical concordance rate in monozygotic twins (about 25%) than dizygotic pairs (about 3%); the French study is exceptional in showing no significant difference between monozygotic and dizygotic twins but critics have argued that this result is within the confidence limits of the other surveys. The relative risk for multiple sclerosis in the monozygotic twin partner of an affected proband is therefore about 190.

Adopted persons who subsequently develop multiple sclerosis, and affected people who have themselves adopted children provide an unusual but informative resource for studying the relative contribution of genes and the environment in the aetiology of multiple sclerosis. Considering those with multiple sclerosis who are adopted before the age of one year, and those with multiple sclerosis who through adoption have non-biological siblings or children, the frequency of multiple sclerosis in non-biological parents, siblings, and children is more or less identical to the population prevalence and lifetime risk for Europeans, and significantly lower than that expected from the study of recurrence risks in the biological relatives of index cases.[64] Half siblings offer yet one more variant on the familial multiple sclerosis theme in that they share a proportion of parental genes and divide into those who are reared together and apart, at least during the period which is thought critical for the development of multiple sclerosis. The age adjusted risk for half siblings is significantly lower than for full siblings and there is no difference in risk for half siblings reared together and apart.[65]

Conjugal pairs with multiple sclerosis who have children provide a special opportunity for assessing the contribution made to susceptibility by genetic factors. Five of 86 offspring from 45 conjugal pairs living in the United Kingdom were shown also to have multiple sclerosis and a further five had either characteristic imaging abnormalities or clinical symptoms consistent with demyelination but did not meet the criteria for clinically definite disease; the recurrence risk (crude 1 in 17: age-adjusted 1 in 5) is obviously much higher than the risk for the children of single affected patients (crude 1 in 200: age adjusted 1 in 50).[66] Conjugal pairs can also be used to assess the influence of environmental factors in determining the onset and course of multiple sclerosis. In the United Kingdom survey, there was no evidence for clinical concordance, clustering at year of onset, or distortion of the expected pattern of age at onset in the second affected spouse from 33 pairs in whom these comparisons could be made.[66] Figure 9.5 summarises these risks.

Markers of genetic susceptibility

The change in recurrence risk seen between twins and first and second degree relatives suggests the independent or epistatic effects of more than one gene; the modest trend for affected pairs to be female hints at a contribution of sex independent of genes; the low concordance rate, even among monozygotic pairs, indicates a significant independent or modifying effect of the environment on expression of genetic susceptibility.

These findings have stimulated attempts to identify and locate the genes which confer susceptibility to the disease. Population studies have shown an association between the class II MHC alleles DR15 and DQ6 and their corresponding genotypes DRB1*1501, DRB5*0101 and DQA1*0102, DQB2*0602.[67] An extensive search, using association and linkage studies, has only yielded additional putative candidate genes in the VH2–5 immunoglobulin heavy chain and the T cell receptor β chain variable regions.[68–71] But the contribution to susceptibility made by the genes which have provisionally been identified, even if their

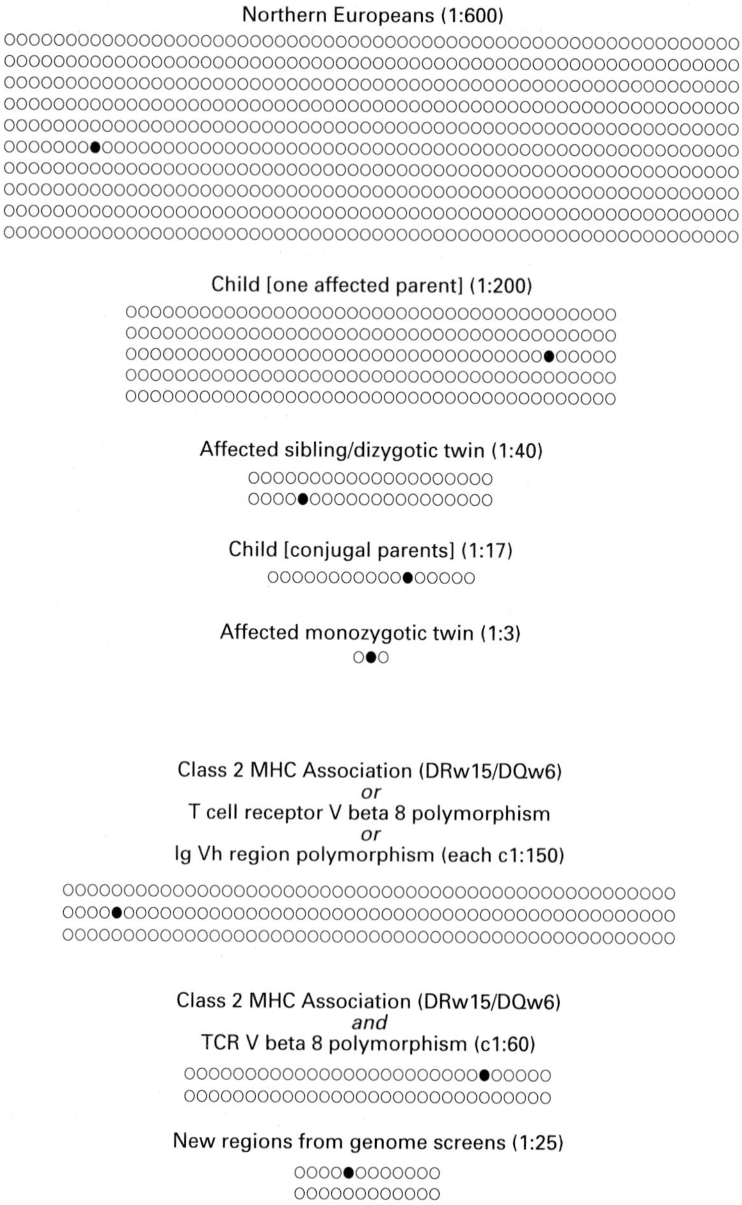

Northern Europeans (1:600)

Child [one affected parent] (1:200)

Affected sibling/dizygotic twin (1:40)

Child [conjugal parents] (1:17)

Affected monozygotic twin (1:3)

Class 2 MHC Association (DRw15/DQw6)
or
T cell receptor V beta 8 polymorphism
or
Ig Vh region polymorphism (each c1:150)

Class 2 MHC Association (DRw15/DQw6)
and
TCR V beta 8 polymorphism (c1:60)

New regions from genome screens (1:25)

Figure 9.5   Scheme to show the reduction in crude risk for multiple sclerosis depending on relation to the proband and the presence of defined susceptibility factors. Comparable age adjusted figures are: children of single affected parents 1 in 50; siblings 1 in 30; children of conjugal pairs 1 in 5; monozygotic twins 1 in 2.

effects are interactive, can only account for a proportion of the increased risk of multiple sclerosis implicated by family studies; and it seems likely that other genes which make an even greater contribution to susceptibility remain to be identified.

Three groups of investigators have now undertaken a systematic search of the genome in an attempt to locate additional susceptibility genes using affected family members—usually identity by descent analysis in sibling pairs. Genotyping was completed on cohorts each of between 75 and 225 families, together involving in excess of 1000 members, for each of between 257–443 microsatellite markers. These markers were chosen to have an average spacing of around 10 cM giving enough power to identify regions encoding a major susceptibility gene; and they are sufficiently polymorphic to make a high proportion of the available families fully informative. Superficially, the results show a disappointing lack of overlap. The importance of HLA is confirmed but of the other new regions of interest, several are clearly unique to each screen and so may be false positives. The regions of interest emerging from the United Kingdom genome screen[72] are 1cen, 5 cen, 6p, 7p, 14q, 17q, 19q, and Xp; they are 2p, 3p, 5p, 11q, and Xp in the Canadian series;[73] and 6p, 7q, 11p, 12q, and 19q in the United States/French survey.[74] Despite inconsistencies between the samples, it remains possible that meta-analysis will provide stronger evidence implicating one or more of these provisional areas of linkage, and the hope is that many of the false positive leads will be eliminated while larger clinical resources are deployed and new strategies pursued for detecting both linkage and new associations within families.

Analysing the epidemiological pattern in multiple sclerosis

The complex interplay of nature and nurture is reflected in the distribution of many diseases; some, such as malaria and the haemoglobinopathies, are reasonably well understood, but factors which determine the geography of complex traits remain much more enigmatic. As parts of Europe and North America were repeatedly surveyed for incidence and prevalence of multiple sclerosis over several decades, neuroepidemiologists began to polarise their views on the emerging patterns around the *race versus place* debate. Especially influential were the serial surveys of stable populations, and the epidemiologically less robust studies of small island populations. It was rapidly pointed out that the gradients in frequency within northern Europe, North America, and Australia compared with other parts of the world implicate an environmental factor in the aetiology of multiple sclerosis which is not ubiquitously distributed. The surveys of multiple sclerosis in northern Europeans migrating west to east provided crucial information implicating the role of environmental factors in shaping the distribution of the disease because, with the exception of Canada, parts of the world colonised from northern Europe show prevalence rates that are lower than in the country of origin. Considerable effort was therefore devoted to a systematic assessment of environmental factors in the hope that a relatively simple causative event would be identified leading to a strategy for eradication of the disease but none was found using either population serology or the most complex methods for virus detection which molecular biology can offer. With time it became clear that more complex patterns of distribution exist within continents and countries, and even across small regions. The evolving epidemiological features of multiple sclerosis made it necessary for epidemiologists to construct ever more elaborate hypotheses to account for the distribution of the disease. Thus there were claims for a role for climate, diet, geomagnetism, and toxins in addition to the infective aetiology.

The migration studies indicate that the risk of multiple sclerosis in a single ethnic group varies with place of residence during a critical period in childhood. However, migration does not just involve the movement of people; gene transfer and population stratification also follow. Failure to define the environmental cause of multiple sclerosis therefore led others to interpret the distribution of multiple sclerosis as a function of genetic susceptibility.[10 75 76] Each of these commentators concluded that multiple sclerosis is to be found where there are northern European genes. It was further suggested that the increased risk of the disease in native people moving out of Africa to the United States correlates with the extent to which white genes are introduced into the black community[77]; and some at least of the affected children of West Indian immigrants to the United Kingdom are known to have white British or Irish ancestors.

The best supporting evidence that markers of susceptibility to multiple sclerosis show much the same geographical patterns as the disease itself comes from the construction of detailed genetic maps which include information on clines for HLA-B7,[78] known to be associated in most populations with an increased risk of multiple sclerosis; presumably the same is true for DR15 and DQ6. As a consequence of sociohistorical events and population migrations, genes with a high frequency in the migrating populations necessarily become concentrated in small isolates whereas others are excluded, thus adding relic groups to the global pattern that exists for many polymorphic genetic markers, and the phenotypically more obvious distributions of language and anthropometrics.

By contrast with the interpretations offered by genetic epidemiologists, backed by evidence from population genetics, environmentalists must still leave the facts to speak for themselves as the case for an environmental agent as the dominant cause of multiple sclerosis remains stubbornly circumstantial. On the basis of the putative epidemic of multiple sclerosis in the Faroes, Kurtzke[7] concludes that multiple sclerosis originated in Scandinavia (central Norway or the south-central lake district of Sweden) in the early 18th century and diffused across the Baltic states and northern Europe including the British Isles over the next 100 years. From there, it was exported to north America and Australasia, to South Africa and Italy. The theme is familiar but whereas for Kurtzke the factors being distributed are germs, for others they are genes.[79]

1 Poser CM, Benedikz J, Hibberd PL. The epidemiology of multiple sclerosis: the Iceland model. Onset-adjusted prevalence rate and other methodological considerations. *J Neurol Sci* 1992;**111**:143–52.

2 Kurtzke JF. A reassessment of the distribution of multiple sclerosis. Part one. *Acta Neurol Scand* 1975;**51**:110–36.

3 Kurtzke JF, A reassessment of the distribution of multiple sclerosis. Part two. *Acta Neurol Scand* 1975;**51**:137–57.

4 Kurtzke JF. Geography in multiple sclerosis. *J Neurol* 1977;**215**:1–26.

5 Bauer HJ. Multiple sclerosis in Europe. Symposium report. *J Neurol* 1987;**234**:195–206.

6 Lauer K, Firnhaber W. *Multiple sclerosis in Europe: an epidemiological update.* Darmstadt: Leuchturm-Verlag/LTV Press, 1994:350.

7 Kurtzke JF. Epidemiologic evidence for multiple sclerosis as an infection. *Clin Microbiol Rev* 1993;**6**:382–427.

8 Robertson NP, Compston DAS. Surveying multiple sclerosis in the United Kingdom. *J Neurol Neurosurg Psychiatry* 1995;**58**:2–6.

9 Rosati G. Descriptive epidemiology of multiple sclerosis in Europe in the 1980s: a critical overview. *Ann Neurol* 1994;**36**(suppl 2):S164–74.

10 Bulman D, Ebers GC. The geography of multiple sclerosis reflects genetic susceptibility. *Journal of Tropical and Geographical Neurology* 1992;**2**:66–72.

11 Hammond SR, McLeod JG, Millingen KS, Stewart-Wynne EG, English D, Holland JT, McCall MG. The epidemiology of multiple sclerosis in 3 Australian cities: Perth, Newcastle, and Hobart. *Brain* 1988;**111**:1–25.

12 Dean G. Annual incidence, prevalence, and mortality of MS in white South African-born and in white immigrants to South Africa. *BMJ* 1967;ii:724–30.

13 Elian M, Dean G. Multiple sclerosis among United Kingdom born children of immigrants from the West Indies. *J Neurol Neurosurg Psychiatry* 987;50:327–32.

14 Elian M, Nightingale S, Dean G. Multiple sclerosis among United Kingdom-born children of immigrants from the Indian subcontinent, Africa, and the West Indies. *J Neurol Neurosurg Psychiatry* 1990;53:906–11.

15 Kurtzke JF, Bui QH. Multiple sclerosis in a migrant population. Half orientals immigrating in childhood. *Ann Neurol* 1980;8:256–60.

16 Alter M, Okihiro M, Rowley W, Morris T. Multiple sclerosis among orientals and caucasians in Hawaii. *Neurology* 1971;21:122–30.

17 Lauer K. The risk of multiple sclerosis in the USA in relation to sociogeographic features: a factor-analytic study. *J Clin Epidemiol* 1994; 47:43–8.

18 Detels R, Brody JF, Edgar AH. Multiple sclerosis among American, Japanese, and Chinese migrants to California and Washington. *J Chron Dis* 1972; 25:3–10.

19 Detels R, Visscher B, Malmgrem RM, Coulson AH, Lucia MV, Dudley JP. Evidence for lower susceptibility to multiple sclerosis in Japanese-Americans. *Am J Epidemiol* 1977;105:303–10.

20 Kuroiwa Y, Shibasaki H, Ikeda M. Prevalence of multiple sclerosis and its north-south gradient in Japan. *Neuroepidemiology* 1983;2:62–9.

21 Alter M, Halpern L, Kurland LT, Bornstein V, Tikva P, Leibowitz U, Silberstein J. Multiple sclerosis in Israel: prevalence among immigrants and native inhabitants. *Arch Neurol* 1962;7:253–63.

22 Alter M, Kahana E, Loewenson R. Migration and risk of multiple sclerosis. *Neurology* 1978;28:1089–93.

23 Kahana E, Zilber N, Abramson JH, Biton Y, Leibowitz Y, Abramsky O. Multiple sclerosis: genetic versus environmental aetiology: epidemiology in Israel updated. *J Neurol* 1994;241:341–6.

24 Kurtzke JF, Kurland LT, Goldberg ID. Mortality and migration in multiple sclerosis. *Neurology* 1971;21:1186–97.

25 Delasnerie-Laupretre N, Alperovitch A. Migration and age at onset of multiple sclerosis: some pitfalls of migrant studies. *Acta Neurol Scand* 1992;85:408–11.

26 Kurtzke JF, Gudmundsson KR, Bergmann S. Multiple sclerosis in Iceland. 1. Evidence of a post-war epidemic. *Neurology* 1982;32:143–50.

27 Cook SD, Gudmundsson G, Benedikz J, Dowling PC. Multiple sclerosis and distemper in Iceland. 1966–78. *Acta Neurol Scand* 1980;61:244–51.

28 Benedikz JG, Magnusson H, Poser CM, Benedikz E, Olafsdottir G, Gudmundsson G. Multiple sclerosis in Iceland 1900–85. *Journal of Tropical Geographical Neurology* 1991;1:16–22.

29 Benedikz JG, Magnusson H, Gudmundsson G. Multiple sclerosis in Iceland, with observations on the alleged epidemic in the Faroe Islands. *Ann Neurol* 1994;36(suppl 2):S175–9.

30 Allison RS. Some neurologic aspects of medical geography. *Proc R Soc Med* 1963;56:71–6.

31 Fog T, Hyllested K. Prevalence of disseminated sclerosis in the Faroes, the Orkneys, and Shetland. *Acta Neurol Scand* 1966;42(suppl 19):9–11.

32 Kurtzke JF, Hyllested K. Multiple sclerosis in the Faroe Islands: 1. Clinical and epidemiological features. *Ann Neurol* 1979;5:6–21.

33 Kurtzke KF, Hyllested K. Multiple sclerosis in the Faroe Islands. II. Clinical update, transmission, and the nature of MS. *Neurology* 1986;36:307–28.

34 Kurtzke JF, Hyllested K. Multiple sclerosis in the Faroe Islands. III. An alternative assessment of the three epidemics. *Acta Neurol Scand* 1987;76:317.

35 Kurtzke JF, Hyllested K. Validity of the epidemics of multiple sclerosis in the Faroe islands. *Neuroepidemiology* 1988;7:190–227.

36 Poser CM, Hibberd PL, Benedicz J, Gudmundsson G. Analysis of the "epidemic" of multiple sclerosis in the Faroe Islands. I. Clinical and epidemiological aspects. *Neuroepidemiology* 1988;7:168–80.

37 Poser CM, Hibberd PL. Analysis of the "epidemic" of multiple sclerosis in the Faroe Islands. II. Biostatistical aspects. *Neuroepidemiology* 1988;7:181–9.

38 Cook SD, Cromarty MB, Tapp W, Poskanzer D, Walker JD, Dowling PC. Declining incidence of multiple sclerosis in the Orkney Islands. *Neurology* 1985;35:545–51.

39 Sheremata WA, Poskanzer DC, Withum DG, MacLeod CL, Whiteside ME. Unusual occurrence on a tropical island of multiple sclerosis [letter]. *Lancet* 1985;ii:618.

40 Weinshenker BG, Bass B, Rice GP, Noseworthy J, Carriere W, Baskerville J, Ebers GC. The natural history of multiple sclerosis: a geographicaly based study. 2. Predictive value of the early clinical course. *Brain* 1989;112:1419–28.

41 Weinshenker BG, Bass B, Rice GP, Noseworthy J, Carriere W, Baskerville J, Ebers GC. The natural history of multiple sclerosis: a geographically based study. 3. Multivariate analysis of predictive factors and models of outcome. *Brain* 1991;114:1045–56.

42 Duquette P, Murray TJ, Pleines J, Ebers GC, Sadovnick D, Weldon P, *et al.* Multiple sclerosis in childhood: clinical profile in 125 patients. *J Pediatr* 1987;3:359–63.

43 Runmarker B, Andersen O. Prognostic factors in a multiple sclerosis incident cohort with 25 years of follow up. *Brain* 1993;116:117–34.

44 Sibley WA, Bamford CR, Clark K, Smith MS, Laguna JF. A prospective study of physical trauma and multiple sclerosis. *J Neurol Neurosurg Psychiatry* 1991;54:584–9.

45 Siva A, Radhakrishnan K, Kurland LT, O'Brien PC, Swanson JW, Rodriguez M. Trauma and multiple sclerosis: a population based cohort study from Olmsted County, Minnesota. *Neurology* 1993;43:1878–82.

46 Baskett PJF, Armstrong R. Anaesthetic problems in multiple sclerosis. *Anaesthesia* 1970;25:397–401.

47 Siemkowicz E. Multiple sclerosis and surgery. *Anaesthesia* 1976;31:1211–6.

48 Sibley, WA, Bamford CR, Clark K. Clinical viral infections and multiple sclerosis. *Lancet* 1985;i:1313–5.

49 Andersen O, Lygner P-E, Berstrom T, Andersson M, Vahlne A. Viral infections trigger multiple sclerosis relapses: a prospective seroepidemiological study. *J Neurol* 1991;240:417–22.

50 Birk K, Ford C, Smeltzer S, Ryan D, Miller R, Rudick RA. The clinical course of multiple sclerosis during pregnancy and the puerperium. *Arch Neurol* 1990;47:738–42.

51 Rouillet E, Verdier-Taillefer M-H, Amarenco P, Gharbi G, Alperovitch A, Marteau R. Pregnancy and multiple sclerosis: a longitudinal study of 125 remittent patients. *J Neurol Nurosurg Psychiatry* 1993;56:1062–5.

52 Worthington J, Jones R, Crawford M, Forti A. Pregnancy and multiple sclerosis—a 3 year prospective study. *J Neurol* 1994;241:228–33.

53 Korn-Lubetzki I, Kahana E, Cooper G, Abramasky O. Activity of multiple sclerosis during pregnancy and puerperium. *Ann Neurol* 1984;16:228–31.

54 Frith JA, McLeod JG. Pregnancy and multiple sclerosis. *J Neurol Neurosurg Psychiatry* 1988;51:495–8.

55 Bernardi S, Grasso MG, Bertollini R, Orzi F, Fieschi C. The influence of pregnancy on relapses in multiple sclerosis: a cohort study. *Acta Neurol Scand* 1991;84:403–6.

56 Runmarker B, Andersen O. Pregnancy is associated with a lower risk of onset and a better prognosis in multiple sclerosis. *Brain* 1995;118:253–61.

57 Sadovnick AD, Baird PA, Ward RH. Multiple sclerosis; updated risks for relatives. *Am J Med Genet* 1988;29:533–41.

58 Robertson NP, Fraser M, Deans J, Clayton D, Compston DAS. Age adjusted recurrence risks for relatives of patients with multiple sclerosis. *Brain* 1996;**119**:449–55.

59 Carton H, Vlietinck R, Debruyne J, De Keyser J, D'Hooghe M-B, Loos R, *et al*. Recurrence risks of multiple sclerosis in relatives of patients in Flanders, Belgium. *J Neurol Neurosurg Psychiatry* 1997;**62**:329–33.

60 Ebers GC, Bulman DE, Sadovnick AD, Paty DW, Warren S, Hader W, *et al*. A population based study of multiple sclerosis in twins. *N Engl J Med* 1986;**315**:1638–42.

61 Sadovnick AD, Armstrong H, Rice GPA, Bulman D, Hashimoto L, Paty DW, *et al*. A population-based study of multiple sclerosis in twins: update. *Ann Neurol* 1993;**33**:281–5.

62 French Research Group on Multiple Sclerosis. Multiple sclerosis in 54 twinships: concordance rate is independent of zygosity. *Ann Neurol* 1992; **32**:724–7.

63 Mumford CJ, NW Wood, HF Kellar-Wood, J Thorpe, Miller D, Compston DAS. The British Isles survey of multiple sclerosis in twins. *Neurology* 1994;**44**:11–5.

64 Ebers GC, Sadovnick AD, Risch NJ. A genetic basis for familial aggregation in multiple sclerosis. *Nature* 1995;**377**:150–1.

65 Sadovnick AD, Ebers GC, Dyment DA, Risch N, the Canadian Collaborative Study Group. Evidence for genetic basis of multiple sclerosis. *Lancet* 1996;**347**: 1728–30.

66 Robertson NP, Clayton D, Fraser MB, Deans J, Compston DAS. Conjugal multiple sclerosis. *Lancet* 1997 (in press).

67 Olerup O, Hillert J. HLA class II-associated genetic susceptibility in multiple sclerosis: a critical evaluation. *Tissue Antigens* 1991;**38**:1–15.

68 Seboun E, Robinson MA, Doolittle TH, Ciulla TA, Kindt TJ, Hauser SL. A susceptibility locus for multiple sclerosis is linked to the T cell receptor β chain complex. *Cell* 1989;**57**:1095–100.

69 Wood NW, Kellar-Wood HF, Holmans P, Clayton D, Robertson N, Compston DAS. The T-cell receptor β locus and susceptibility to multiple sclerosis. *Neurology* 1995;**45**:1859–63.

70 Walter MA, Gibson WT, Ebers GC, Cox DW. Susceptibility to multiple sclerosis is associated with the proximal immunoglobulin heavy chain region. *J Clin Invest* 1991;**87**:1266–73.

71 Wood N, Sawcer SJ, Kellar-Wood H, Holmans P, Clayton D, Robertson N, Compston DAS. A susceptibility gene for multiple sclerosis linked to the immunoglobulin heavy chain variable region. *J Neurol* 1995;**242**:677–82.

72 Sawcer S, Jones HB, Feakes R, Gray J, Smaldon N, Chataway J, *et al*. A genome screen in multiple sclerosis reveals susceptibility loci on chromosome 6p21 and 17q22. *Nat Genet* 1996;**13**:464–8.

73 Ebers GC, Kukay K, Bulman D, Sadovnick AD, Rice G, Anderson C, *et al*. A full genome search in multiple sclerosis. *Nat Genet* 1996;**13**:472–6.

74 The Multiple Sclerosis Genetics Group. A complete genomic screen for multiple sclerosis underscores a role for the major histocompatibility complex. *Nat Genet* 1996;**13**:469–71.

75 Davenport CB. Multiple sclerosis from the standpoint of geographic distribution and race. *Arch Neurol* 1922;**8**:51–8.

76 Sutherland JM. Observations on the prevalence of multiple sclerosis in northern Scotland. *Brain* 1956;**79**:635–54.

77 Chakraborty R, Kamboh, MI, Nwankwo M, Ferrell RE. Caucasian genes in American blacks: new data. *Am J Hum Genet* 1992;**50**:145–55.

78 Cavalli-Sforza LL, Menozzi P, Piazza A. *The history and geography of human genes*. Princeton: Princeton Universty Press, 1994:541.

79 Poser CM. The dissemination of multiple sclerosis: a Viking saga? A historical essay. *Ann Neurol* 1994;**36**(suppl 2):S231–43.

10 The Dementias

CORNELIA van DUIJN

> - Dementia is a rapidly growing health problem in all the developed world.
> - Cross-cultural studies show variation in rates of dementia but have not yet thrown much light on causation.
> - In recent years there has been considerable progress in unravelling the genetics of dementia.
> - In contrast, powerful environmental determinants of dementia have yet to be identified.
> - Studies of gene–environment interaction may offer the best prospect for understanding aetiology.

Dementia is an important cause of disability in elderly people. Given the increase in the proportion of elderly people in most countries, the number of patients with dementia will rise and the care of these patients will have a growing impact on the healthcare system and society. The past decade has seen many successes in epidemiological studies of the aetiology of chronic disorders including cardiovascular disease, cancer, and osteoporosis. In this review, new developments in the epidemiology of the dementias are discussed. Descriptive studies of the occurrence of dementia across different populations and time periods as well as studies of risk factors for dementia are reviewed. Dementia is a syndrome that can be caused by many conditions. As Alzheimer's disease is the predominant cause of dementia, accounting for at least half of the cases in most populations, epidemiological research has focused on this disorder.

Geographical trends

Cross cultural comparison of the occurrence of disease has led to important clues to risk factors implicated in chronic disorders such as cardiovascular disease and cancer. The number of epidemiological studies on dementia is still small compared with these other chronic disorders. However, several community based studies have considered the *prevalence* of dementia—that is, the number of patients with dementia alive in a defined population and time frame. These studies have been reviewed recently.[1-3] An important limitation of prevalence studies is that differences in occurrence and survival of disease in a population cannot be distinguished. They are of little value when comparing the risk of dementia across populations. Community based studies of the *incidence* of dementia—that is, the number of patients that are newly diagnosed in a defined population and time frame—are to be preferred.

At present, there are only a limited number of such studies available.[4-17] Table 10.1 shows their general characteristics. In all studies, the diagnosis of dementia and Alzheimer's disease was in accordance with currently accepted criteria.[18-19] Figures 10.1 and 10.2 present age specific incidence rates of dementia and Alzheimer's disease. Up to the age of 75 years, there is little evidence for a large variation in dementia and Alzheimer's disease between studies. The incidence of Alzheimer's disease seems to be increased in the east Boston study[16]; however, this may be explained by the fact that the diagnosis of Alzheimer's disease was based primarily on psychometric testing.[4] There is considerable variation in the incidence of dementia and Alzheimer's disease

Table 10.1   General characteristics of community based studies on the age specific incidence of dementia and Alzheimer's disease

	No of subjects studied	Period of follow up (y)	Age range (y)
Europe:			
Lundby, Sweden[5]	3563	25	All
Gothenburg, Sweden[4]	385	4–5	70–79
Mannheim, Germany[13]	1912	7–8	65+
Bordeaux, France[14]	2792	3	65+
Liverpool, UK[8]	1070	3	65+
Nottingham, UK[10]	1042	4	65+
Cambridge, UK[15]	1195	2·4	75+
London, UK[12]	705	3	65+
North America:			
Rochester, USA[11]★	55000	25	All
New York, USA[6]	488	8	75+
Framingham, USA[9]	2117	10	65+
East Boston, USA[16]†	2312	4·3	65+
Asia:			
Hisayama, Japan[17]	828	7	65+
Beijing, China[7]	1090	3	60+

★Although based on a medical register, the coverage of this register is such that it may be considered community based.
†Incidence is estimated based on a sample of 642 patients who received detailed clinical examination.

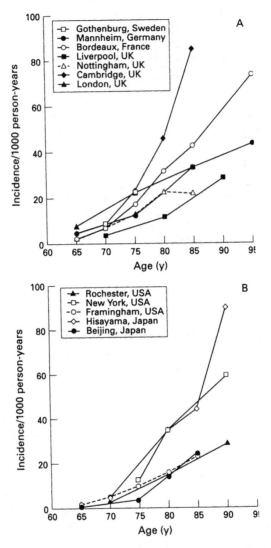

Figure 10.1 Comparison of age specific incidence of dementia in community based studies in Europe (A) and elsewhere (B).

between populations after the age of 75 years, which is not likely to be a result of differences in diagnostic criteria given the lack of variation up to the age of 75 years. However, the few subjects at risk in some studies, methodological problems related to non-response, competing mortality, and comorbidity complicating the

212

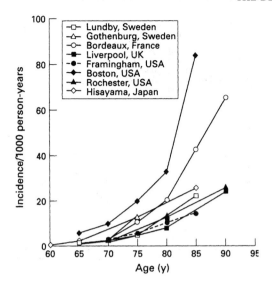

Figure 10.2 Comparison of age specific incidence of Alzheimer's disease in community based studies.

diagnosis make it doubtful whether these variations truly reflect a difference in incidence of dementia between populations.

There is some evidence that the relative proportion attributed to the most common subtypes, Alzheimer's disease and vascular dementia, differs between populations.[20] In studies of Caucasian populations from Europe and North America, over 50% of all patients with dementia were attributed to Alzheimer's disease compared with only 12–30% to vascular causes.[20] In Asian populations, vascular dementia was found to be underlying the dementia in up to 60% of the patients.[20] In the two Japanese studies of incident patients, vascular dementia constituted 40% and 60% of all dementia.[7 17] As the incidence of Alzheimer's disease was similar across populations, this suggests that the incidence of vascular dementia may be increased in Asian populations.[7 17] It may be speculated that genetic or environmental factors underlie the differences in incidence of vascular dementia across populations. However, there are two important considerations. Firstly, vascular dementia may be underestimated in Caucasian populations as some prevalence studies in Caucasians have reported a proportion of vascular dementia up to 50%.[4 21] Secondly, an intrinsic problem when comparing different populations for the relative proportion of Alzheimer's disease and vascular dementia is the fact that the diagnosis of vascular dementia is based on the presence of dementia and cerebrovascular disease. The diseases may be related, but no causal relation between the vascular pathology and the dementia can be established in patients. This may bias the comparison of populations with different rates of vascular disease, as this would inevitably predict a higher proportion of vascular dementia in populations with a higher rate of vascular disease. As the clinical diagnosis of Alzheimer's disease is based on the exclusion of other causes of dementia, including vascular dementia, this may also affect the prevalence of Alzheimer's disease. Similar problems relate to the comparison of the frequency of subtypes of dementia between Caucasian and Afro-American populations. Because of the higher frequency of hypertension and stroke in Afro-Americans, an increased proportion of the vascular and the mixed Alzheimer and vascular type of dementia[22] would be expected. In the absence of biological markers and unequivocal clinical or morphological criteria, cross cultural comparisons of the risk of subtypes of dementia will be difficult to interpret.

Time trends

Variation in incidence of dementia over time within a population may lead to hypotheses about environmental risk factors. Again, studies of the *prevalence* of dementia are less informative for this as they may be biased by differences in survival. Despite the lack of specific treatment, survival of patients may have improved.[5 23 24] There are only two long term follow up studies available which have monitored *incidence* of dementia over time. Data on the incidence of senile dementia over a 25 year period (1947–72) are available from a study conducted in Lundby, Sweden.[5] In this study, there was no evidence for a trend over time. Data on incidence collected in Rochester, Minnesota in the period 1960–84 suggested that changes in incidence of dementia may have occurred.[11] A higher incidence of dementia was found in the earliest (1960–4) as well as the latest (1980–4) period studied and was found to be limited to the very old. However, the increased awareness of dementing illness in the past decade may have influenced rates of diagnosis in the later period.[11] So far, studies of trends in the incidence of dementia over time have yielded few clues about the aetiology of the disease.

Clinical characteristics

Clinical epidemiological studies in patients with heterogeneous disorders, such as Alzheimer's disease and other subtypes of dementia, may lead to advances in the understanding of the pathophysiology and open new leads to interventions that slow the progression of disease. Further, subtyping of dementias according to aetiology is important in establishing prognosis as well as for selection of homogeneous case series for clinical trials. The existence of subgroups may be explored by studies on clinical and pathological characteristics and survival of patients. Here, the characteristics of the two most common subtypes of dementia, Alzheimer's disease and vascular dementia, are discussed.

Alzheimer's disease

Neuropathological features of Alzheimer's disease comprise neuritic plaques, amyloid angiopathy, neuronal loss, and neurofibrillary tangles. Amyloid fibrils composed of the amyloid protein (A4 protein) make up the core of the neuritic plaques. Neurofibrillary tangles consist of intraneuronal paired helical filaments, which are in part composed of altered forms of the microtubule associated protein tau. Although clinically Alzheimer's disease is a diagnosis by exclusion of other causes of dementia,[18 19] the disease is characterised by an impaired learning ability, a decline in language function, and deterioration of visuospatial skills.[25] Calculation, abstraction, and judgement are often affected, the onset of the disease is insidious, and in the early stages, changes in personality are common.[18 19 25]

Although the origin of the disease is unknown in most patients, there are known gene mutations that may cause an early onset form of Alzheimer's disease. Mutations in the β amyloid precursor protein (APP) gene on chromosome 21 have been found in a few families, which cause an autosomal dominant form of early onset Alzheimer's disease (onset < 55 years).[26] Recently, two homologous genes—presenilin 1 (PS-1) on chromosomes 14 and presenilin 2 (PS-2) on chromosome 1—have been identified that lead to familial autosomal dominant forms of early onset Alzheimer's disease (onset age between 30–55 years and 50–70 years respectively).[27–29] The ε4 allele of the apolipoprotein E gene on chromosome 19 (APOE*4) has been shown to be associated with an increased risk for late onset[30 31] as well as early onset Alzheimer's disease.[32 33]

Patients with dementia have a reduced life expectancy compared with the general population and other institutionalised patients.[23][24][34][35] Among patients with Alzheimer's disease, there are major differences in mortality.[34] The wide range in survival may in part be explained by differences in duration of disease at entry into the study. A meta-analysis of community, clinic, and nursing home based studies on survival showed mortality to be increased in men.[34] However, studies of prevalent cases may be biased as patients who die early in the course of disease are less likely to be included in the study, resulting in an overestimation of survival. Survival in incident cases has been considered in four community based studies.[4][6][8][24] Survival was significantly worse in male patients with Alzheimer's disease in a study in Rochester,[24] but not in others.[4][6] However, the small sample size hampers the interpretation of the latter studies. Findings in the Rochester study suggest that five year survival (period 1975–84) decreases with age of onset of disease from 84% in patients with an onset at or before 69 years to 81% in patients with an onset between 70 and 79 years and to 40% in patients with an onset after 80 years.[24] However, the reduced survival in elderly patients may be a consequence of the reduced life expectancy in the late onset patients. After adjusting for the higher life expectancy in younger patients, a study conducted in New York (the Bronx), suggested that the risk of mortality increased with decreasing age of onset of disease.[6] This finding suggests that an earlier onset of disease may be more malignant.

Alzheimer's disease is often accompanied by the development of extrapyramidal symptoms, myoclonus, psychosis, seizures, aphasia, and primitive reflexes.[36-39] Several studies have shown that patients developing one of these symptoms tend to deteriorate to specific cognitive and functional end points more rapidly than those without these symptoms.[36-40] It is not clear at present whether these symptoms reflect a clinical subgroup of patients with Alzheimer's disease or whether they are merely markers of disease progression. The finding of an increasing frequency of these symptoms during the course of disease is compatible with the view that these factors are markers of disease progression.[36] On the other hand, the frequency of myoclonus and aphasia early in the course of disease is increased in patients of families in which Alzheimer's disease is linked to a mutation on chromosome 14.[41-43] This suggests that these clinical features reflect different aetiology. The ongoing dissection of Alzheimer's disease by its

216

genetic causes may yield important information on the origin and relevance of concomitant pathology in Alzheimer's disease.

Little is known of the relation between genetic factors and mortality in patients with Alzheimer's disease. The number of patients with dominant mutations is small, which complicates studies on the relation of these mutations to survival. However, it has been shown that patients of families in which Alzheimer's disease is inherited as an autosomal dominant disorder have, in general, a worse progression.[44] Findings on APOE*4 have been controversial. One study reported no association between survival and clinical characteristics,[45] whereas other studies suggest that APOE*4 is associated with a slower progression and prolonged survival in patients with Alzheimer's disease.[46-48] The $\varepsilon2$ allele of apolipoprotein E (APOE*2) has been associated with an increased mortality in one study,[48] but this finding remains to be confirmed.

Vascular dementia

Vascular dementia is a syndrome that may be caused by several vascular lesions, including ischaemic, hypoxic, and haemorrhagic brain damage.[25] The clinical diagnosis requires the presence of (a) dementia, (b) cerebrovascular disease evidenced by neuroimaging and by neurological symptoms, and (c) a temporal relation between the vascular disease and dementia.[25] Vessel occlusion seems to be the most common pathology underlying vascular dementia.[25]

Several clinical subtypes of vascular dementia have been recognised, including multi-infarct dementia, lacunar state, and Binswanger's disease.[25] Diagnosis of these subtypes of vascular dementia syndromes has been facilitated by the progress in neuroimaging.[49] Clinical-epidemiological studies with MRI are likely to play an important part in separating clinically and aetiologically relevant subgroups, especially in combination with genetic studies. Thus far, genetic and MRI studies have been successful in unravelling the aetiology of cerebral autosomal dominant arteriopathy with subcortical infarcts and leuko-encephalopathy (CADASIL).[50 51] This is an inherited disease associated with dementia, stroke and transient ischaemic attacks, migraine with aura, and mood disorders.[50 51] Abnormalities on MRI are found in the subcortical white matter and basal ganglia and can be detected before the clinical expression of the

217

disease.[50][51] Molecular research suggests that CADASIL is linked to a gene on chromosome 19.[50]

Studies on the survival of patients have consistently shown a reduced life expectancy for patients with vascular dementia compared with the general population. Survival is worse than in patients with Alzheimer's disease.[21][23][34][35][39] The number of studies on predictors of survival for vascular dementia is still small, but male sex,[39][52] low education,[52] advanced disability,[39] and primitive reflexes[39] have been associated with poorer prognosis.

Risk factors

Most studies of risk factors for dementia have focused on the commonest subtype, Alzheimer's disease. Studies conducted before 1991 have been reviewed and collaboratively reanalysed by the EURODEM Risk Factors Research Group.[53-60] Here, the findings of more recent studies will be evaluated in the light of this reanalysis. However, it is important to realise that most studies were based on the comparison of prevalent cases of Alzheimer's disease with control subjects.[53] Such studies are prone to various types of bias. Selection bias may have occurred due to mortality in patients related to the risk factor studied. Assessment of exposure to the risk factor has often been based on information from surrogates, which may introduce error. Further, differential misclassification in exposure to risk factors between cases and controls may have occurred, as informants of patients may have been better at recalling exposures than controls. The relation of most risk factors for Alzheimer's disease remains to be confirmed in follow up studies of incident patients, in which the exposure state is measured before the onset of disease.

Age and sex

The risk of dementia and Alzheimer's disease increases strongly with age (see figs 10.1 and 10.2),[1-3] suggesting that genetic and environmental factors which influence aging of the brain may play an important part. Two studies of the incidence of Alzheimer's disease found that the disease occurred more often in women than men,[5][17] but most studies show a similar incidence in men and women.[4][8][9][11][14] Vascular dementia has been found to be more frequent in men than women,[4 14 17] which probably reflects the higher frequency of vascular disease in men. The incidence of vascular dementia in men and women increased with age in the long term follow up study conducted in Lundby.[5] By contrast, an increase in incidence of vascular dementia with age was found only in women in the study conducted in the Bordeaux area in France.[14] However, the number of patients studied was small.

Genetic risk factors

Alzheimer's disease aggregates within families of patients with early and late onset of disease.[54] Several genes (APP, PS-1, PS-2) have been identified that are involved in the autosomal dominant forms of early onset Alzheimer's disease.[26-29] However, the role of these genes in late onset Alzheimer's disease, which concerns the vast majority of patients in the population, is limited. In the patients with late onset disease, the APOE gene on chromosome 19 seems to play a part.[30-32] Other forms of dementia including vascular dementia,[61 62] Lewy body disease,[63] and Creutzfeldt-Jakob disease[64] have also been associated with APOE*4. Further, APOE*4 has been associated with decreased cognitive function and increased rates of cognitive decline in the general population.[65-68]

Despite the fact that many studies have consistently shown an increased risk of Alzheimer's disease for APOE*4 carriers,[69] some questions remain to be clarified to identify clinically relevant risk groups. There is still controversy about whether the risk associated with the APOE*4 allele may be modified by sex,[70-72] ethnicity,[73-75] age,[72 76] or family history of dementia.[33 72 77] Although findings of two studies are compatible with modification of the risk of Alzheimer's disease for APOE*4 carriers by sex,[70 72] one study failed to show evidence for interaction.[71] Among African and Afro-American populations, the risk associated with APOE*4 is unclear as a lack of association between APOE*4 and the risk of Alzheimer's disease has been found in some studies[73 75] but not in others.[74] Several studies found the relation between APOE*4 and Alzheimer's disease to be absent in the very elderly patients.[76 78] Some studies have suggested that the strongest effect of APOE*4 occurs in those with a positive family history.[33 77] A meta-analysis on the modification of the strength of association between APOE*4 and the risk of Alzheimer's disease by age and family history of dementia showed that the APOE*4 allele frequency was highest among patients with familial Alzheimer's disease, the APOE*4 frequency being 0·48 (95% confidence interval (95% CI): 0·45–0·51) in those with late onset and 0·42 (95% CI: 0·36–0·48) in those with early onset of disease.[69] The APOE*4 allele frequency was significantly higher in patients with late onset sporadic Alzheimer's disease (APOE*4 frequency: 0·37; 95% CI: 0·35–0·39) than in patients with early onset sporadic disease (APOE*4 frequency: 0·28; 95% CI: 0·23–0·33).[69] This finding suggests that the risk of disease may be modified by age in patients with sporadic Alzheimer's disease.

Another issue that remains to be resolved is the association of Alzheimer's disease with the APOE*2 allele. Several studies noted a lower frequency of the APOE*2 allele in patients with Alzheimer's disease, suggesting that there may be a protective effect of APOE*2.[32 79] However, an increased risk for carriers of APOE*2 was found in an Italian,[80] a Dutch,[48] and an Afro-American population.[74] There are several possible explanations for the differences in association between Alzheimer's disease and APOE*2 across populations, including linkage disequilibrium with another gene and modification by other genetic and environmental factors.[48] The discrepancies may also be a result of the reduced survival of patients with APOE*2.[48] As most studies were based on prevalent cases, APOE*2 carriers may have been selectively removed from the patient series over time. This may have resulted in an apparent decrease of the APOE*2 allele frequency. In a similar way, the increased survival for patients with Alzheimer's disease with APOE*4 that has been found in some studies may have led to an overrepresentation of APOE*4 carriers in patients with Alzheimer's disease.[46-48] Although it is unlikely that the relation between APOE*4 and Alzheimer's disease can be explained fully by survival effects, reduced mortality in APOE*4 carriers may have led to an overestimation of the risk of Alzheimer's disease associated with the APOE*4 allele.[48]

The mechanism through which APOE affects the risk of Alzheimer's disease and other types of dementia remains to be elucidated. The APOE*4 allele has been implicated in various aspects of Alzheimer's disease pathology including β A4 amyloid deposition in senile plaques as well as in microtubule instability and paired helical filament formation.[30 81] APOE*4 has also been shown to increase the risk of atherosclerosis, which may explain its association with vascular dementia.

Down's syndrome

The increased risk of Alzheimer's disease in people with Down's syndrome has long been recognised. Alzheimer pathology has been found in most elderly patients with Down's syndrome.[82] When pooling and reanalysing the early case-control studies, there was considerable evidence for familial aggregation of Down's syndrome and both early and late onset Alzheimer's disease,[54] but recent studies of patients with Alzheimer's disease have failed to show a significant association.[83-89] However, the negative findings may be a result of the low statistical power of individual studies.

As the frequency of Alzheimer's disease in the population is considerably higher than the frequency of Down's syndrome, studies of family history of dementia in patients with Down's syndrome have a higher statistical power. Although the early studies on family history did not yield consistent results,[90 91] a recent study has shed new light on this issue.[92] The study showed an increased risk of dementia in mothers of patients with Down's syndrome, but not in fathers, suggesting that non-dysjunction of chromosomes in the mother may play a part in familial aggregation of Down's syndrome and Alzheimer's disease.[92] The risk of dementia in mothers was increased only when the mother was younger than 35 years old at the birth of the child with Down's syndrome.[92] This finding suggests that the association is not explained by an increased risk of non-dysjunction with advanced maternal age but that other factors are involved. Because familial aggregation of Down's syndrome and Alzheimer's disease has been found to be strongest in those with a positive family history, it is possible that genetic factors may be implicated.[93]

Parkinson's disease and Lewy body disease

Alzheimer's disease, Parkinson's disease, and Lewy body disease share several pathological features. The Lewy body and Alzheimer pathology can be found in each of these disorders. Dementia, a cardinal feature of Alzheimer's disease and Lewy body dementia, is often found in patients with Parkinson's disease.[25 94] There is some evidence for a common genetic origin of these disorders. Early studies were compatible with familial aggregation of Alzheimer's disease and Parkinson's disease,[54] being strongest in the families of patients with a positive family history of dementia.[93] Although more recent studies failed to confirm familial aggregation of these disorders,[83-85 88 89] the results of molecular genetic research suggest that they may have a common genetic origin. An increased risk of both Alzheimer's disease and Lewy body dementia has been associated with the APOE gene.[30-33] [63] In recent studies, CYP2D6B, a gene that has been associated with Parkinson's disease and Lewy body disease, has also been associated with the Lewy variant of Alzheimer's disease and with synaptic pathology in Alzheimer's disease.[95 96] It is not yet clear whether any of these findings may explain familial aggregation of these disorders.

Maternal age at birth

As a corollary of the findings on Down's syndrome and family history of Down's syndrome, parental age has been studied as a potential risk factor for Alzheimer's disease. The findings are inconsistent. Some studies have suggested an association with late maternal age,[55 85 88] some found a significant increase in risk for young maternal[55 97] and young paternal age,[86 97] and some found no evidence for an association at all.[55 89] Although young parental age has been associated with a moderate increase in risk of Down's syndrome, it seems unlikely that the strong association of Alzheimer's disease with young maternal and paternal age can be explained by an increase in risk of chromosome 21 non-dysjunction in meiosis at an early age.[55]

Head trauma

Repeated head trauma in boxers has been associated with dementia pugilistica. The similarity in pathology of dementia pugilistica to the Alzheimer pathology has led to the hypothesis of a common pathogenesis of Alzheimer's disease and dementia. Early epidemiological studies were remarkably consistent in showing that patients were more often exposed to head trauma in the past than were controls, although the differences were not always significant.[56] Of the recent studies, three reported a significant increased risk of Alzheimer's disease after head trauma,[89 98 99] and four did not.[83-85 88] Studies of the history of head trauma have all been hampered by recall bias. Relatives of patients may have been more likely to remember head injuries that occurred in the past than relatives of controls. One prospective follow up study based on data obtained from the Rochester medical records showed only a slight and non-significant increase in risk.[56] However, a recent study suggests that the association may be modified by the presence of the APOE*4 allele.[100] An increased risk of Alzheimer's disease after head trauma was only found in carriers of the APOE*4 allele.[100] Any bias in recalling head trauma would be expected to be independent of APOE genotype and this finding, if confirmed, lends strong support to a relation between head trauma and Alzheimer's disease in the subgroup of cases who are APOE*4 carriers. Regarding the biological mechanism, recent experimental studies suggested that the expression of β amyloid and interleukin 1 are increased after head trauma and that head trauma may be related to Alzheimer's disease through the induction of an acute phase response.[101]

Depression

Early studies suggested that a history of depression may be a risk factor for Alzheimer's disease.[58] The risk of Alzheimer's disease increased for those treated for depression 10 years or more before the first symptoms of dementia, suggesting that the depression was not simply a consequence of the dementia.[58] A similar association was present in a follow up study, in which the history of depression before the onset of disease was assessed from medical records.[58] Two recent studies showed no relation between depression and Alzheimer's disease,[83 89] but another reported a non-significant increase in risk of Alzheimer's disease in subjects with a history of depression in the previous three years.[86] Familial aggregation of depression has been reported in patients with Alzheimer's disease and a positive family history of dementia.[102] This suggests that genetic factors may underlie the relation.[102] However, it remains to be excluded that depression is merely an early sign of Alzheimer pathology.

Thyroid disease

There is some evidence from the early studies of risk factors for Alzheimer's disease for an increased risk of disease in patients with hypothyroidism.[57] Further, an association between Alzheimer's disease and autoimmune thyroid disease has been reported in Down's syndrome and familial Alzheimer's disease.[103 104] None of the recent studies has confirmed the association with thyroid disease.[83 88 89] However, these studies were based on data from informants. One study on the history of thyroid disease based on medical records suggested that the risk of Alzheimer's disease was decreased for patients with Graves' disease, whereas there was a non-significant increase in risk for patients with myxoedema.[105] These findings and their pathophysiological importance remain to be clarified.

Vascular factors

In recent years, the interest in vascular causes of dementia has increased, partly because there may be opportunities for prevention and treatment for this type of dementia. By definition, vascular disease and its risk factors must be present in patients with vascular dementia.[25] Factors that have been implicated in the risk of vascular dementia include hypertension, diabetes mellitus, and cardiovascular disease.[106] The mechanism through which these factors lead to dementia is unclear. Vascular factors may also be involved in Alzheimer's disease.[106] However, their role is difficult to quantify as patients with vascular disease are less likely to be diagnosed as cases of Alzheimer's disease.[18 19] White matter lesions have been found in increased frequency in patients with Alzheimer's disease in some studies but not in others.[107 108] Although these lesions have been associated with atherosclerosis,[109] they are not specific and may reflect cerebral atrophy and amyloid angiopathy in patients with Alzheimer's disease.[107 108] There is evidence from one MRI study that suggests that arteriolosclerosis may be specific for patients with late onset Alzheimer's disease.[108]

Anti-inflammatory drugs

From experimental studies, there is increasing evidence that acute and chronic inflammatory processes play an important part in the pathophysiology of Alzheimer's disease.[110 111] Novel findings that may have clinical relevance are the inverse relations between Alzheimer's disease and past use of anti-inflammatory drugs and with rheumatoid arthritis, a disorder for which these drugs are often prescribed.[84 89 112–114] As the only follow up study failed to show a relation between rheumatoid arthritis and Alzheimer's disease,[115] a possible protective effect of anti-inflammatory drugs remains to be clarified. Preliminary evidence showing that cognitive decline may be less in subjects taking indomethacin than in control subjects, indicates that further studies may be of interest.[116]

Oestrogen replacement therapy

Oestrogen may be implicated in Alzheimer's disease in several ways. Improvement of cerebral blood flow, direct stimulation of neurons, development of gliacytes, and suppression of apolipoprotein E have been suggested.[117] However, findings of epidemiological studies have been controversial. One study, based on computerised pharmaceutical records, did not show evidence for a relation,[118] whereas two studies based on anamnestic data suggested a protective effect of oestrogen replacement therapy.[119 120] There are important methodological problems which make the interpretation of the latter studies difficult. In one, a follow up study, based on direct interviews before onset of disease, the diagnosis of Alzheimer's disease at follow up depended on mortality records.[119] Mortality records have been shown to be unreliable for the ascertainment of patients with Alzheimer's disease. In the other study, the history of oestrogen use was obtained from informants for cases of Alzheimer's disease but from the control women directly.[120] Lack of knowledge of the use of oestrogens by the informant may explain part of the inverse relation found. Although some experimental studies on oestrogen suggest a beneficial effect,[117] there is no convincing evidence from epidemiological studies confirming such a role of oestrogen in Alzheimer's disease.

Smoking history

Early epidemiological studies suggested an inverse association between Alzheimer's disease and history of smoking,[59] but recent studies have yielded equivocal results. The association between smoking and Alzheimer's disease was found to be absent in three studies,[88 89 121] inverse in two,[122 123] and positive in one.[86] The inverse association seemed to be related to social class in one study.[123] The results of a recent meta-analysis were compatible with a decreased risk of Alzheimer's disease in smokers.[124] There is some evidence that genetic factors, including the APOE gene, may alter the association between smoking and Alzheimer's disease.[93 125] The inverse relation between smoking and Alzheimer's disease was found to be limited to those with the APOE*4 allele that had a positive family history.[93 125] However, modification of the relation between smoking and Alzheimer's disease by APOE has not been confirmed in other studies.[126]

Experimental studies of rats and rabbits have suggested that nicotine may improve memory and cognition.[127] Moreover, blockade of nicotinic receptor function may produce a significant cognitive impairment in humans[128] and clinical trials have suggested that nicotine and nicotine derivatives may improve information processing and attention in patients with Alzheimer's disease.[129 130] However, there was no evidence for improvements in memory or cognition.[129 130] This suggests that nicotine or its derivates modifies a rather limited spectrum of the clinical course of the disease.

Most studies of Parkinson's disease have also reported an inverse association with smoking.[131] By contrast with the findings on Alzheimer's disease and Parkinson's disease, the risk of vascular dementia was found to be increased for subjects that smoked,[106] suggesting a different effect of smoking in these disorders, rather than a general mechanism between smoking and dementia.

Alcohol

There was no evidence for an increase in risk of Alzheimer's disease in people with a moderate alcohol intake in a reanalysis of early case-control studies of Alzheimer's disease.[59] Also, no relation was found between alcohol consumption and Alzheimer's disease in two recent studies including one follow up study.[89 122] These findings should be treated with caution. Cases with higher alcohol intake may have been excluded when applying the criteria for probable or possible Alzheimer's disease,[18 19] leading to an underestimation in risk. Indeed, alcohol misuse has been associated with a significant increased risk of dementia[132] and Alzheimer's disease[85] in two population based studies.

Occupational exposure

Findings on occupational exposure to solvents have been controversial. No significant increased risk for occupational exposure to solvents and lead was found when pooling the early studies.[60] However, in the pooled analysis frequency of exposure was low and exposure definition was imprecise.[60] Two recent case-control studies have reported an association with occupational exposures.[89 133] In one study, an increased risk of Alzheimer's disease was found for subjects exposed to glues and pesticides.[89] Another study suggested a statistically significant increase in risk of Alzheimer's disease for men exposed to solvents such as benzene, toluene, phenols, alcohols, and ketones.[133] Studies on subjects exposed occupationally to solvents have suggested that risk of neurological symptoms may be modified by heavy alcohol consumption.[134] Whether the increased risk for Alzheimer's disease depends on the alcohol consumption or some other occupational exposure is not known at present.

Aluminum

There has been extensive debate on the question whether aluminum is implicated in the aetiology of Alzheimer's disease. The initial epidemiological studies were instigated in response to the finding of aluminum in neuritic plaques and tangle-bearing neurons. However, more recent studies of the association between aluminum and the Alzheimer pathology have yielded contradicting results.[135] On the other hand, there is growing evidence from experimental studies that aluminum may influence the conformation of both amyloid and neurofibrillary tangles.[136-138]

Follow up studies of the presence of Alzheimer pathology in the brains of patients who were on dialysis and exposed to high doses of aluminum have not been conclusive.[139 140] Epidemiological studies on the association between aluminum in drinking water and the risk of Alzheimer's disease have been reviewed recently.[141] With the exception of one study,[88] findings have been consistent in suggesting an increased risk of Alzheimer's disease with increasing aluminum concentration in drinking water.[141 142] However, the possibility of bias in present studies still outweighs the evidence for causal inference.[141] Studies that have considered the role of aluminum products such as antacids and antiperspirants have yielded equivocal results.[84 89] Supporting a role of aluminum in Alzheimer's disease was the finding of a lower level of cognitive functioning among miners treated with aluminum powder[143] and the finding of a slower progression of the disease in patients with Alzheimer's disease treated with aluminum chelating drugs.[144]

Despite the strong evidence from experimental studies that aluminum may be implicated in the Alzheimer pathology and progression of the disease, there are many questions to be answered from an epidemiological point of view. An issue that complicates the interpretation of the negative studies is the possibility that the effect of aluminum may depend on an interaction with other environmental factors. For instance, the risk of Alzheimer's disease associated with aluminum in drinking water may be influenced by the pH[142] or the presence of silicon.[145] Aluminum concentrations in serum and bone from cases of Alzheimer's disease are not raised suggesting that aluminum exposure and absorption is similar in patients with Alzheimer's disease and controls.[146 147] However, it is conceivable that genetic factors[148] or other (patho)physiological factors (for example, head trauma) may enable aluminum to enter the brain. Thus the increase in risk of Alzheimer's disease associated with aluminum may be present only in a subgroup of patients. These are issues that can only be considered in large scale epidemiological studies.

Education

It has been suggested that highly educated subjects have a lower risk of Alzheimer's disease and other types of dementia.[149] However, this finding was based on prevalent cases.[149] Two community based studies of incident cases failed to show an association of education with risk of Alzheimer's disease, suggesting that survival and selection bias may explain the earlier results.[150 151] Recent studies have produced conflicting results. Higher educational attainment was associated with an increased mortality[152] but a less severe stage of disease at the time of presentation in patients with Alzheimer's disease.[153] A relation between risk of vascular dementia and lower education levels was also found in a study of incident cases.[151] This finding may be explained by the relation between low socioeconomic class and vascular disease.

Discussion

By contrast with epidemiological studies of other chronic disorders, cross cultural studies have not led to important clues to the aetiology of dementia or any of its subtypes. There may be differences in the risk of vascular dementia between populations, but comparative studies of geographical and time trends are difficult to interpret because of the lack of biological markers and unique clinical features for the subtypes of dementia. Cross cultural comparison of studies of Alzheimer's disease showed no evidence for the existence of risk factors that are to be found predominantly in some populations but not in others. The risk factors for Alzheimer's disease seem to be ubiquitous.

Aetiological studies have uncovered some putative risk factors for Alzheimer's disease. There is growing evidence that several disorders including Down's syndrome, Parkinson's disease, depression, head injury, and perhaps thyroid disease may be associated with an increase in the risk of Alzheimer's disease. Familial aggregation of Alzheimer's disease with Down's syndrome, depression, and perhaps Parkinson's disease suggests that there may be a common genetic factor underlying these disorders in at least a subgroup of patients. As to environmental factors, the influence of alcohol and smoking is still controversial. Given the widespread exposure to aluminum through food products and drinking water, the relation between aluminum and Alzheimer's disease deserves further attention.

Epidemiological research on Alzheimer's disease is far from its limits. Most studies of risk factors for this disease have been small, whereas risk factors were rare.[53] The validity of studies has been compromised by anamnestic data collected through surrogate informants. Long term follow up studies, that are currently ongoing, will overcome these problems. Non-response, competing mortality, and comorbidity complicating the diagnosis, in particular in elderly people, will be challenges to overcome in these studies. However, advances in epidemiological research will not depend only on improved methodology. Recent epidemiological studies have led to preliminary findings of a protective effect of anti-inflammatory drugs and perhaps oestrogen replacement therapy that may prove to be of clinical relevance. Progress in the understanding of the genetics of Alzheimer's disease and other types of dementia has opened new possibilities for epidemiological studies on the risk associated with these genetic factors. Firstly, the risk of Alzheimer's disease associated with the various genetic factors identified including APOE remains to be quantified in follow up studies of incident cases. Secondly, the possibility of interaction between genetic and environmental risk factors needs to be studied, as the strength of association between an environmental factor and the risk of disease may depend on the presence of a genetic factor.[93] Conversely, the effect of the genetic factor on the risk of

Alzheimer's disease may be conditional on the presence of other genetic and environmental risk factors.[93] For APOE, there is some evidence for synergistic effects of APOE*4, head trauma, and cholesterol and antagonistic effects of APOE*4 and smoking with regard to the risk of Alzheimer's disease.[72 100 125] Interaction of APOE with other possible risk factors including vascular factors needs to be studied further. As pathological and molecular biological research proceeds, Alzheimer's disease and other types of dementia are likely to be dissected further into aetiologically relevant subgroups.

CMvD is supported by grants of the Netherlands Organization for Scientific Research (NWO) and the Netherlands Institute for Health Sciences (NIHES). ACJW Janssens and AJC Slooter are acknowledged for helpful discussions of the manuscript.

1 Hofman A, Rocca WA, Brayne C, et al. The prevalence of dementia in Europe: a collaborative study of 1980–1990 findings. Int J Epidemiol 1991;20:381–90.

2 Rocca WA, Hofman A, Brayne C, et al. Frequency and distribution of Alzheimer's disease in Europe: a collaborative study of 1980–1990 findings. Ann Neurol 1991;381:381–90.

3 Breteler MMB, Claus JJ, van Duijn CM, et al. Epidemiology of Alzheimer's disease. Epidemiol Rev 1992;14:59–82.

4 Nilsson LV. Incidence of severe dementia in an urban sample followed from 70–79 years of age. Acta Psychiatr Scand 1984;70:478–86.

5 Rorsman B, Hagnell O, Lanke J. Prevalence and incidence of senile and multi-infarct dementia in the Lundby study: a comparison of the time periods 1947–1957 and 1957–1972. Neuropsychobiology 1986;15:122–9.

6 Aronson MK, Ooi WL, Geva DL. Dementia. Age-dependent incidence, prevalence and mortality in the old old. Arch Intern Med 1991;151:989–92.

7 Li G, Shen YC, Chen CH, et al. A three-year follow-up study of age-related dementia in an urban area of Beijing. Acta Psychiatr Scand 1991;83:99–104.

8 Copeland JRM, Davidson IA, Dewey ME, et al. Alzheimer's disease, other dementia, depression and pseudo-dementia: prevalence, incidence and three-year outcome in Liverpool. Br J Psychiatry 1992;161:230–9.

9 Bachman DL, Wolf PA, Linn RT, et al. Incidence of dementia and Alzheimer's disease in a general population: the Framingham Study. Neurology 1993;43:515–9.

10 Morgan K, Lilley JM, Arie T, et al. Incidence of dementia in a representative British sample. Br J Psychiatry 1993;163:467–70.

11 Kokmen E, Beard CM, O'Brien PC, et al. Is the incidence of dementing illnes changing? A 25-year time trend study in Rochester, Minnesota (1960–1984). Neurology 1993;43:1887–92.

12 Boothby H, Blizard R, Livingston G, Mann AH. The Gospel Oak Study stage III: the incidence of dementia. Psychobiol Med 1994;24:89–95.

13 Bickle H, Cooper B. Incidence and relative risk of dementia in an urban elderly population. Findings of a prospective field study. Psychobiol Med 1994;24:179–92.

14 Letenneur L, Commenges RD, Dartigues JF, Saberger-Gateau P. Incidence of dementia and Alzheimer's disease in elderly community residents of south-western France. Int J Epidemiol 1994;23:1256–61.

15 Paykel ES, Brayne C, Huppert F, *et al*. Incidence of dementia in a population older than 75 years in the United Kingdom. *Arch Gen Psychiatry* 1994;**51**:325–32.

16 Hebert LE, Scherr PA, Beckett LA, *et al*. Age-specific incidence of Alzheimer's disease in a community population. *JAMA* 1995;**273**:1354–9.

17 Yoshitake T, Kiyohara Y, Kato I, *et al*. Incidence and risk factors of vascular dementia and Alzheimer's disease in a defined elderly Japanese population. The Hisayama study. *Neurology* 1995;**45**:1161–8.

18 American Psychiatric Association. Diagnostic and statistical manual of mental disorders. 3rd ed revised. Washington, DC: American Psychiatric Association, 1980.

19 McKhann G, Drachman D, Folstein M, *et al*. Clinical diagnosis of Alzheimer's disease: report of the NINCDS-ADRDA Work Group under the auspices of Department of Health and Human Services Task Force on Alzheimer's disease. *Neurology* 1984;**34**:39–44.

20 Jorm AF. Cross-national comparison of the occurrence of Alzheimer's disease and vascular dementia. *Eur Arch Psychiatry Clin Neurosci* 1991;**240**:218–22.

21 Skoog I, Nilsson L, Palmertz B, *et al*. A population-based study of dementia in 85-year-olds. *N Engl J Med* 1993;**328**:153–8.

22 Heyman A, Fillenbaum G, Prosnitz B, *et al*. Estimated prevalence of dementia among elderly black and white community residents. *Arch Neurol* 1991;**48**:594–8.

23 Rorsman B, Hagnell O, Lanke J. Prevalence of age psychosis and mortality among aged psychotics in the Lundby study. *Neuropsychology* 1985;**13**:167–72.

24 Beard CM, Kokmen E, O'Brien PC, Kurland LT. Are patients with Alzheimer's disease surviving longer in recent years? *Neurology* 1994; **44**:1869–71.

25 Cumlings CL. The failing brain. *Lancet* 1995;**345**:1481–9.

26 Goate A, Chartier-Harlin M-C, Mullan M, *et al*. Seggregation of a missense mutation in the amyloid precursor protein gene with familial Alzheimer's disease. *Nature* 1991;**349**:704–6.

27 Sherrington R, Rogaev EI, Liang Y, *et al*. Cloning of a gene bearing missense mutations in early-onset familial Alzheimer's disease. *Nature* 1995; **375**:754–60.

28 Levy-Lahad E, Wasco W, Poorkaj P, *et al*. Candidate gene for the chromosome 1 familial Alzheimer's disease locus. *Science* 1995;**269**:973–7.

29 Rogaev EI, Sherrington R, Rogaeva EA, *et al*. Familial Alzheimer's disease in kindreds with a missense mutation in a gene on chromosome 1 related to the Alzheimer's disease type 3 gene. *Nature* 1995;**376**:775–8.

30 Strittmatter WJ, Saunders AM, Schmechel D, *et al*. Apolipoprotein E: high avidity binding to beta-amyloid and increased frequency of type 4 allele in late-onset familial Alzheimer's disease. *Proc Natl Acad Sci USA* 1993;**90**:1977–81.

31 Saunders AM, Strittmatter WJ, Schmechel D, *et al*. Association of apolipoprotein E allele epsilon 4 with late-onset familial and sporadic Alzheimer's disease. *Neurology* 1993;**43**:1467–72.

32 Chartier-Harlin MC, Parfitt M, Legrain S, *et al*. Apolipoprotein E, ε4 allele as a major risk factor for sporadic early and late-onset form of Alzheimer's disease: analysis of the 19q13·2 chromosomal region. *Hum Molec Genet* 1994;**3**:569–74.

33 Van Duijn CM, de Knijff P, Cruts M, *et al*. Apolipoprotein E ε4 allele in a population-based study of early-onset Alzheimer's disease. *Nature Genet* 1994;**7**:74–8.

34 Van Dijk PTM, Dippel DWJ, Habbema JDF. Survival of patients with dementia. *J Am Geriatr Soc* 1991;**39**:603–10.

35 Katzman R, Hill LR, Yu ES, *et al*. The malignancy of dementia. Predictors of mortality in clinically diagnosed dementia in a population survey of Shanghai, China. *Arch Neurol* 1994;**51**:1220–5.

36 Chen JY, Stern Y, Sano M, Mayeux R. Cumalative risk of developing extrapyramidal signs, psychosis, or myoclonus in the course of Alzheimer's disease. *Arch Neurol* 1991;**48**:1141–3.

37 Risse SC, Lampe TH, Bird TD, *et al*. Myoclonus, seizures, and paratonia in Alzheimer's disease. *Alzheimer Dis Assoc Disord* 1990;**4**:217–25.

38 Knesevich JW, Toro FR, Morris JC, *et al*. Aphasia, family history, and the longitudinal course of senile dementia of the Alzheimer type. *Psychiatry Res* 1985;**14**:255–63.

39 Molsa PK, Martilla RJ, Rinne UK. Long term survival and predictors of mortality in Alzheimer's disease and multi-infarct dementia. *Acta Neurol Scand* 1995;**91**:159–64.

40 Stern Y, Mayeux R, Chen JY, *et al*. Predictors of mortality in Alzheimer's disease. *Ann Neurol* 1989;**26**:132.

41 Kennedy AM, Neuman SK, Frackowiak RS, *et al*. Chromosome 14 linked familial Alzheimer's disease. A clinico-pathological study of a single pedigree. *Brain* 1995;**118**:185–205.

42 Haltia M, Viitanen M, Sulkava R, *et al*. Chromosome 14-encoded Alzheimer's disease: genetic and clinicopathological description. *Ann Neurol* 1994;**36**:362–7.

43 Lampe TH, Bird TD, Nochlin D, *et al*. Phenotype of chromosome 14-linked familial Alzheimer's disease in a large kindred. *Ann Neurol* 1994;**36**:368–78.

44 Farrer LA, Cupples LA, Van Duijn CM, *et al*. Rate of progression of Alzheimer's disease is associated with genetic risk. *Arch Neurol* 1995;**52**:918–23.

45 Corder EH, Saunders AM, Strittmatter WJ, *et al*. Apolipoprotein E, survival in Alzheimer's disease patients, and the competing risks of death and Alzheimer's disease. *Neurology* 1995;**45**:1323–8.

46 Basun H, Grut M, Winblad B, Lannfelt L. Apolipoprotein epsilon 4 allele and disease progression in patients with late-onset Alzheimer's disease. *Neurosci Lett* 1995;**183**:32–4.

47 Frisoni GB, Govoni S, Geroldi C, *et al*. Gene dose of the epsilon 4 allele of apolipoprotein E and disease progression in sporadic late-onset Alzheimer's disease. *Ann Neurol* 1995;**37**:596–604.

48 Van Duijn CM, de Knijff P, Wehnert A, *et al*. The apolipoprotein E $\varepsilon2$ allele is associated with an increased risk of early-onset Alzheimer's disease and a reduced survival. *Ann Neurol* 1995;**37**:605–10.

49 Pantoni L, Garcia JH. The significance of white matter abnormalities 100 years after Binswanger's report. *Stroke* 1995;**26**:1293–301.

50 Tournier-Lasserve E, Joutel A, Melki J, *et al*. Cerebral autosomal dominant arteriopathy with subcortical infarcts and leukoencephalopathy maps to chromosome 19q12. *Nature Genet* 1993;**3**:256–9.

51 Chabriat H, Vahedi K, Iba-Zizen MT, *et al*. Clinical spectrum of CADASIL: a study of 7 families. Cerebral autosomal dominant arteriopathy with subcortical infarcts and leukoencephalopathy. *Lancet* 1995;**346**:934–9.

52 Hier DB, Wallace JD, Gorelick PB, *et al*. Predictors of survival in clinically diagnosed Alzheimer's disease and multi-infarct dementia. *Arch Neurol* 1989;**46**:1213–6.

53 Van Duijn CM, Stijnen T, Hofman A. Risk factors for Alzheimer's disease: overview of the collaborative re-analysis of case-control studies. *Int J Epidemiol* 1991;**20** (suppl):S4–12.

54 Van Duijn CM, Clayton D, Chandra V, et al. Familial aggregation of Alzheimer's disease and related disorders: a collaborative re-analysis of case-control studies. Int J Epidemiol 1991;20 (suppl):S13–20.

55 Rocca WA, van Duijn CM, Chandra V, et al. Maternal age and Alzheimer's disease: a collaborative re-analysis of case-control studies. Int J Epidemiol 1991;20 (suppl):S21–7.

56 Mortimer JA, van Duijn CM, Chandra V, et al. Head trauma as a risk factor for Alzheimer's disease: a collaborative re-analysis of case-control studies. Int J Epidemiol 1991;20 (suppl):S28–35.

57 Breteler MMB, van Duijn CM, Chandra V, et al. Medical history and the risk of Alzheimer's disease: a collaborative re-analysis of case-control studies. Int J Epidemiol 1991;20(suppl):S36–42.

58 Jorm AF, van Duijn CM, Chandra V, et al. Psychiatric history and related exposures as risk factors for Alzheimer's disease: a collaborative re-analysis of case-control studies. Int J Epidemiol 1991;20(suppl):S43–7.

59 Graves AB, van Duijn CM, Chandra V, et al. Alcohol and tobacco consumption as risk factors for Alzheimer's disease: a collaborative re-analysis of case-control studies. Int J Epidemiol 1991;20(suppl):S48-S57.

60 Graves AB, van Duijn CM, Chandra V, et al. Occupational exposures to solvent and lead as risk factors for Alzheimer's disease: a collaborative re-analysis of case-control studies. Int J Epidemiol 1991;20 (suppl):S58–61.

61 Shimano H, Murase T, Ishibashi S, et al. Plasma apolipoproteins in patients with multi-infarct dementia. Atherosclerosis 1989;79:257–60.

62 Frisoni GB, Geroldi C, Bianchetti A, et al. Apolipoprotein E epsilon 4 allele frequency in vascular dementia and Alzheimer's disease. Stroke 1994;25:1703–4.

63 St Clair D, Norrman J, Perry R, et al. Apolipoprotein E epsilon 4 allele frequency in patients with Lewy body dementia, Alzheimer's disease and age-matched controls. Neurosci Lett 1994;176:45–6.

64 Amouyel P, Vidal O, Launay JM, Laplanche JL. The apolipoprotein E alleles as major susceptibility factors for Creutzfeldt-Jakob disease. The French Research Group on Epidemiology of Human Spongiform Encephalopathies. Lancet 1994;344:1315–8.

65 Reed T, Carmelli D, Swan GE, et al. Lower cognitive performance in normal older adult male twins carrying the apolipoprotein E epsilon 4 allele. Arch Neurol 1994;51:1189–92.

66 Feskes E, Havekes LM, Kalmijn S, et al. Apolipoprotein E4 allele and congnitive decline in elderly men. BMJ 1994;309:1202–6.

67 Henderson AS, Easteal S, Jorm AF, et al. Apolipoprotein E allele E4, dementia and cognitive decline in a population sample. Lancet 1995; 346:1387–90.

68 Petersen RC, Smith GE, Ivnik RJ, et al. Apolipoprotein E status as a predictor of the development of Alzheimer's disease in memory-impaired individuals. JAMA 1995;273:1274–8.

69 Van Gool WA, Evenhuis HM, van Duijn CM, on behalf of the Dutch Study Group on Down's Syndrome and Ageing. A case-control study of apolipoprotein E genotypes in Alzheimer's disease with Down's syndrome. Ann Neurol 1995;38;225–30.

70 Payami H, Montee KR, Kaye JA, et al. Alzheimer's disease, apolipoprotein E4, and gender (letter). JAMA 1994;271:1316–7.

71 Corder EH, Saunders AM, Strittmatter WJ, et al. The apolipoprotein E E4 allele and sex-specific risk of Alzheimer's disease. JAMA 1995;273:373–74.

72 Jarvik GP, Wijsman EM, Kukull WA, et al. Interactions of apolipoprotein E genotype, total cholesterol level, age, and sex in prediction of Alzheimer's disease: a case-control study. Neurology 1995;45:1092–6.

73 Hendrie HC, Hall KS, Hui S, *et al*. Apolipoprotein E genotypes and Alzheimer's disease in a community study of elderly African Americans. *Ann Neurol* 1995;**37**:118–20.

74 Maestre G, Ottman R, Stern Y, *et al*. Apolipoprotein E and Alzheimer's disease: ethnic variation in genotypic risks. *Ann Neurol* 1995;**37**:254–59.

75 Hendrie HC, Hall KS, Hui S, *et al*. Apolipoprotein E genotypes and Alzheimer's disease in a community study of elderly African Americans. *Ann Neurol* 1995;**37**:118–20.

76 Rebeck GW, Perls TT, West HL, *et al*. Reduced apolipoprotein epsilon 4 allele frequency in the oldest old Alzheimer's patients and cognitively normal individuals *Neurology* 1994;**44**:1513–6.

77 Lannfelt L, Lilius L, Nastase M, *et al*. Lack of association between apolipoprotein E allele epsilon 4 and sporadic Alzheimer's disease. *Neurosci Lett* 1994;**169**:175–8.

78 Sobel E, Louhija J, Sulkava R, *et al*. Lack of association of apolipoprotein E allele epsilon 4 with late-onset Alzheimer's disease among Finnish centenarians. *Neurology* 1995;**45**:903–7.

79 Corder EH, Saunders AM, Risch NJ, *et al*. Protective effect of apolipoprotein E type 2 allele for late onset Alzheimer disease. *Nature Genet* 1994;**7**:180–4.

80 Sorbi S, Nacmias B, Forleo P, *et al*. ApoE allele frequencies in Italian sporadic and familial Alzheimer's disease. *Neurosci Lett* 1994;**177**:100–2.

81 Strittmatter WJ, Roses AD. Apolipoprotein E and Alzheimer disease. *Proc Natl Acad Sci USA* 1995;**92**:4725–7.

82 Holland AJ, Oliver C. Down's syndrome and the links with Alzheimer's disease. *J Neurol Neurosurg, Psychiatry* 1995;**59**:111–4.

83 Mendez MF, Underwood KL, Zander BA, *et al*. Risk factors in Alzheimer's disease: a clinicopathologic study. *Neurology* 1992;**42**:770–5.

84 Li G, Shen YC, Li YT, *et al*. A case-control study of Alzheimer's disease in China. *Neurology* 1992;**42**:1481–8.

85 Fratiglioni L, Ahlbom A, Viitanen M, Winblad B. Risk factors for late-onset Alzheimer's disease: a population-based, case-control study. *Ann Neurol* 1993;**33**:258–66.

86 Prince M, Cullen M, Mann A. Risk factors for Alzheimer's disease and dementia: a case-control study based on the MRC elderly hypertension trial. *Neurology*, 1994 **44**:97–104.

87 Sadovnick AD, Yee IM, Hirst C. The rate of the Down syndrome among offspring of women with Alzheimer disease. *Psychiatric Genetics* 1994;**4**:87–9.

88 Forster DP, Newens AJ, Kay DW, Edwardson JA. Risk factors in clinically diagnosed presenile dementia of the Alzheimer type: a case-control study in northern England. *J Epidemiol Comm Health* 1995;**49**:253–8.

89 The Canadian Study of Health and Aging: risk factors for Alzheimer's disease in Canada. *Neurology* 1994;**44**:2073–80.

90 Yatham LN, McHale PA, Kinsella A. Down syndrome and its association with early-onset Alzheimer's disease. *Acta Psychiatry Scand* 1988;**77**:38–41.

91 Berr C, Borghi E, Rethore MO, *et al*. Absence of familial association between dementia of the Alzheimer type and Down syndrome. *Am J Med Genet* 1989;**33**:545–50.

92 Schupf N, Kapell D, Lee JH, *et al*. Increased risk of Alzheimer's disease in mothers of adults with Down's syndrome. *Lancet* 1994;**344**:353–6.

93 Van Duijn CM, Clayton DG, Chandra V, *et al*. Interaction between genetic and environmental risk factors for Alzheimer's disease: a reanalysis of case-control studies. *Genet Epidemiol* 1994;**11**:539–51.

94 De Vos RA, Jansen EN, Stam FC *et al*. 'Lewy body disease': clinico-pathological correlations in 18 consecutive cases of Parkinson's disease with and without dementia. *Clin Neurol Neurosurg* 1995;**97**:13–22.

95 Saitoh T, Xia Y, Chen X, et al. The CYP2D6B mutant allele is overrepresented in the Lewy body variant of Alzheimer's disease. Ann Neurol 1995;37:110–2.

96 Chen X, Xia Y, Alford M, et al. The CYP2D6B allele is associated with a milder synaptic pathology in Alzheimer's disease. Ann Neurol 1995;38:653–8.

97 Farrer LA, Cupples LA, Connor L, et al. Association of decreased paternal age and late-onset Alzheimer's disease. Arch Neurol 1991;48:599–604.

98 Mayeux R, Ottman R, Tang MX, et al. Genetic susceptibility and head injury as risk factors for Alzheimer's disease among community-dwelling elderly persons and their first-degree relatives. Ann Neurol 1993;33:494–501.

99 Rasmussen DX, Brandt J, Martin DB, Folstein MF. Head injury as a risk factor in Alzheimer's disease. Brain Injury 1995;9:213–9.

100 Mayeux R, Ottman R, Maestre G, et al. Synergistic effects of traumatic head injury and apolipoprotein-epsilon 4 in patients with Alzheimer's disease. Neurology 1995;45:555–7.

101 Roberts GW, Gentleman SM, Lynch A, et al. Beta amyloid protein deposition in the brain after severe head injury: implications for the pathogenesis of Alzheimer's disease. J Neurol Neurosurg Psychiatry 1994;57:419–25.

102 Luchins DJ, Cohen D, Hanrahan P, et al. Are there clinical differences between familial and non-familial Alzheimer's disease? Am J Psychiatry 1992;149:1023–7.

103 Percy ME, Dalton AJ, Markovic VD, et al. Autoimmune thyroiditis associated with mild "subclinical" hypothyroidism in adults with Down syndrome: a comparison of patients with and without manifestations of Alzheimer's disease. Am J Med Genet 1990;36:140–54.

104 Ewins DL, Rossor MN, Butler J, et al. Association between autoimmune thyroid disease and familial Alzheimer's disease. Clin Endocrinol 1991;35:93–6.

105 Kokmen E, Beard CM, Chandra V, et al. The association between Alzheimer's disease and thyroid disease in Rochester, Minnesota. Neurology 1991;41:1745–7.

106 Skoog I. Risk factors for vascular dementia: a review. Dementia 1994;5:137–44.

107 Verny M, Duyckaerts C, Pierot L, Hauw JJ. Leuko-araiosis. Dev Neurosci 1991;13:245–50.

108 Scheltens P, Barkhof F, Valk J, et al. White matter lesions on magnetic resonance imaging in clinically diagnosed Alzheimer's disease. Evidence for heterogeneity. Brain 1992;115:735–48.

109 Bots ML, van Swieten JC, Breteler MMB, et al. Cerebral white matter lesions and atherosclerosis in the Rotterdam Study. Lancet 1993; 341:1232–7.

110 Dash PK, Moore AN. Enhanced processing of APP induced by IL-1 beta can be reduced by indomethacin and nordihydroguaiaretic acid. Biochem Biophys Res Commun 1995;208:542–8.

111 Brugg B, Dubreuil YL, Huber G, et al. Inflammatory processes induce beta-amyloid precursor protein changes in mouse brain. Proc Natl Acad Sci USA 1995;92:3032–5.

112 Breitner JC, Gau BA, Welsh KA, et al. Inverse association of anti-inflammatory treatments and Alzheimer's disease: initial results of a co-twin control study. Neurology 1994;44:227–32.

113 Lucca U, Tettamanti M, Forloni G, Spagnoli A. Nonsteroidal anti-inflammatory drug use in Alzheimer's disease. Biol Psychiatry 1994;36:854–6.

114 Andersen K, Launer LJ, Ott A, *et al.* Do nonsteroidal anti-inflammatory drugs decrease the risk for Alzheimer's disease? The Rotterdam Study. *Neurology* 1995;45:1441–5.

115 Beard CM, Kokmen E, Kurland T. Rheumatoid arthritis and susceptibility to Alzheimer's disease. *Lancet* 1991;337:1426,

116 Rich JB, Rasmusson DX, Folstein MF, *et al.* Nonsteroidal anti-inflammatory drugs in Alzheimer's disease. *Neurology* 1995;45:51–5.

117 Honjo H, Tanaka K, Kashiwagi T, *et al.* Senile dementia-Alzheimer's type and estrogen. *Horm Metab Res* 1995;27:204–7.

118 Brenner DE, Kukull WA, Stergachis A, *et al.* Postmenopausal estrogen replacement therapy and the risk of Alzheimer's disease: a population-based case-control study. *Am J Epidemiol* 1994;140:262–7.

119 Paganini-Hill A, Henderson VW. Estrogen deficiency and risk of Alzheimer's disease in women. *Am J Epidemiol* 1994;140:256–61.

120 Henderson VW, Paganini-Hill A, Emanuel CK, *et al.* Estrogen replacement therapy in older women. Comparisons between Alzheimer's disease cases and nondemented control subjects. *Arch Neurol* 1994;51:896–900.

121 Hebert LE, Scherr PA, Beckett LA, *et al.* Relation of smoking and alcohol consumption to incident Alzheimer's disease. *Am J Epidemiol* 1992;135:347–55.

122 Brenner DE, Kukull WA, van Belle G, *et al.* Relationship between cigarette smoking and Alzheimer's disease in a population-based case-control study. *Neurology* 1993;43:293–300.

123 Letenneur L, Dartigues JF, Commenges D, *et al.* Tobacco consumption and cognitive impairment in elderly people. A population-based study. *Ann Epidemiol* 1994;4:449–54.

124 Lee PN. Smoking and Alzheimer's disease: a review of the epidemiological evidence. *Neuroepidemiology* 1994;13:131–44.

125 Van Duijn CM, Havekes LM, Van Broeckhoven C, *et al.* Apolipoprotein E genotype and association between smoking and early onset Alzheimer's disease. *BMJ* 1995;310:627–31.

126 Plassman BL, Helms MJ, Welsh KA, *et al.* Smoking, Alzheimer's disease, and confounding with genes (letter). *Lancet* 1995;345:387.

127 Nitta A, Katono Y, Itoh A, *et al.* Nicotine reverses scopolamine-induced impairment of performance in passive avoidance task in rats through its action on the dopaminergic neuronal system. *Pharmacol Biochem Behav* 1995;49:807–12.

128 Newhouse PA, Potter A, Corwin J, Lenox R. Age-related effects of the nicotinic antagonist mecamylamine on cognition and behavior. *Neuropsychopharmacology* 1994;10:93–107.

129 Jones GM, Sahakian BJ, Levy R, *et al.* Effects of acute subcutaneous nicotine on attention, information processing and short-term memory in Alzheimer's disease. *Psychopharmacology* 1992;108:485–94.

130 Wilson AL, Langley LK, Monley J, *et al.* Nicotine patches in Alzheimer's disease: pilot study on learning, memory, and safety. *Pharmacol Biochem Behav* 1995;51:509–14.

131 Morens DM, Grandinetti A, Reed D, *et al.* Cigarette smoking and protection from Parkinson's disease: false association or etiologic clue? *Neurology* 1995;45:1041–51.

132 Saunders PA, Copeland JR, Dewey ME, *et al.* Heavy drinking as as risk factor for depression and dementia in elderly men. Finding from the Liverpool longitudinal study. *Br J Psychiatry* 1991;159:213–6.

133 Kukull WA, Larson EB, Bowen JD, *et al.* Solvent exposure as a risk factor for Alzheimer's disease: a case-control study. *Am J Epidemiol* 1995;141:1059–71.

134 Edling C, Ekberg K, Ahlborg G Jr, *et al.* Long-term follow-up of workers exposed to solvents. *Br J Ind Med* 1990;47:75–82.

135 Landsberg JP, McDonald B, Watt F. Absence of aluminium in neuritic plaque cores in Alzheimer's disease. *Nature* 1992;**360**:65–8.

136 Kawahara M, Muramoto K, Kobayashi K, *et al*. Aluminum promotes the aggregation of Alzheimer's amyloid beta-protein in vitro. *Biochem Biophys Res Commun* 1994;**198**:531–5.

137 Fasman GD, Perczel A, Moore CD. Solubilization of beta-amyloid-(1-42)-peptide: reversing the beta-sheet conformation induced by aluminum with silicates. *Proc Natl Acad Sci USA* 1995;**92**:369–71.

138 Scott CW, Fieles A, Sygowski LA, Caputo CB. Aggregation of tau protein by aluminum. *Brain Res* 1993;**628**:77–84.

139 Candy JM, McArthur FK, Oakley AE, *et al*. Aluminium accumulation in relation to senile plaque and neurofibrillary tangle formation in the brains of patients with renal failure. *J Neurol Sci* 1992;**107**:210–8.

140 Harrington CR, Wischik CM, McArthur FK, *et al*. Alzheimer's-disease-like changes in tau protein processing: association with aluminium accumulation in brains of renal dialysis patients. *Lancet* 1994;**343**:993–7.

141 Doll R. Review: Alzheimer's disease and environmental survival bias. *Age Ageing* 1993;**22**:138–53.

142 Jacqmin H, Commenges D, Letenneur L, *et al*. Components of drinking water and risk of cognitive impairment in the elderly. *Am J Epidemiol* 1994;**139**:48–57.

143 Rifat SL, Eastwood MR, McLachlan DR, *et al*. Effect of exposure of miners to aluminium powder. *Lancet* 1990;**336**:1162–5.

144 Crapper McLachlan DR, Dalton AJ, Kruck TP, *et al*. Intramuscular desferrioxamine in patients with Alzheimer's disease. *Lancet* 1991; **337**:1304–8.

145 Edwardson JA, Moore PB, Ferrier IN, *et al*. Effect of silicon on gastrointestinal absorption of aluminium. *Lancet* 1993;**342**:211–2.

146 O'Mahony D, Denton J, Templar J, *et al*. Bone aluminium content in Alzheimer's disease. *Dementia* 1995;**6**:69–72.

147 Zapatero MD, Garcia de Jalon A, Pascual F, *et al*. Serum aluminium levels in Alzheimer's disease and senile dementias. *Biol Trace Elem Res* 1995;**47**:235–40.

148 Fosmire GJ, Focht SJ, McClearn GE. Genetic influences on tissue deposition of aluminum in mice. *Biol Trace Elem Res* 1993;**37**:115–21.

149 Katzman R. Education and the prevalence of dementia and Alzheimer's disease. *Neurology* 1993;**43**:13–20.

150 Beard CM, Kokmen E, Offord KP, Kurland LT. Lack of association between Alzheimer's disease and education, occupation, marital status, or living arrangement. *Neurology* 1992;**42**:2063–8.

151 Cobb JL, Wolf PA, Au R, *et al*. The effect of education on the incidence of dementia and Alzheimer's disease in the Framingham Study. *Neurology* 1995;**45**:1707–12.

152 Stern Y, Tang MX, Denaro J, Mayeux R. Increased risk of mortality in Alzheimer's disease patients with more advanced educational and occupational attainment. *Ann Neurol* 1995;**37**:590–5.

153 Moritz DJ, Petitti DB. Association of education with reported age of onset and severity of Alzheimer's disease at presentation: implications for the use of clinical samples. *Am J Epidemiol* 1993;**137**:456–62.

Index

Page numbers printed in **bold** type refer to figures; those in *italic* to tables

Coventry University